C Bigelow

Sexual pathology

A practical and popular review of the principal diseases of the reproductive organs

C Bigelow

Sexual pathology

A practical and popular review of the principal diseases of the reproductive organs

ISBN/EAN: 9783742821645

Manufactured in Europe, USA, Canada, Australia, Japa

Cover: Foto ©Lupo / pixelio.de

Manufactured and distributed by brebook publishing software (www.brebook.com)

C Bigelow

Sexual pathology

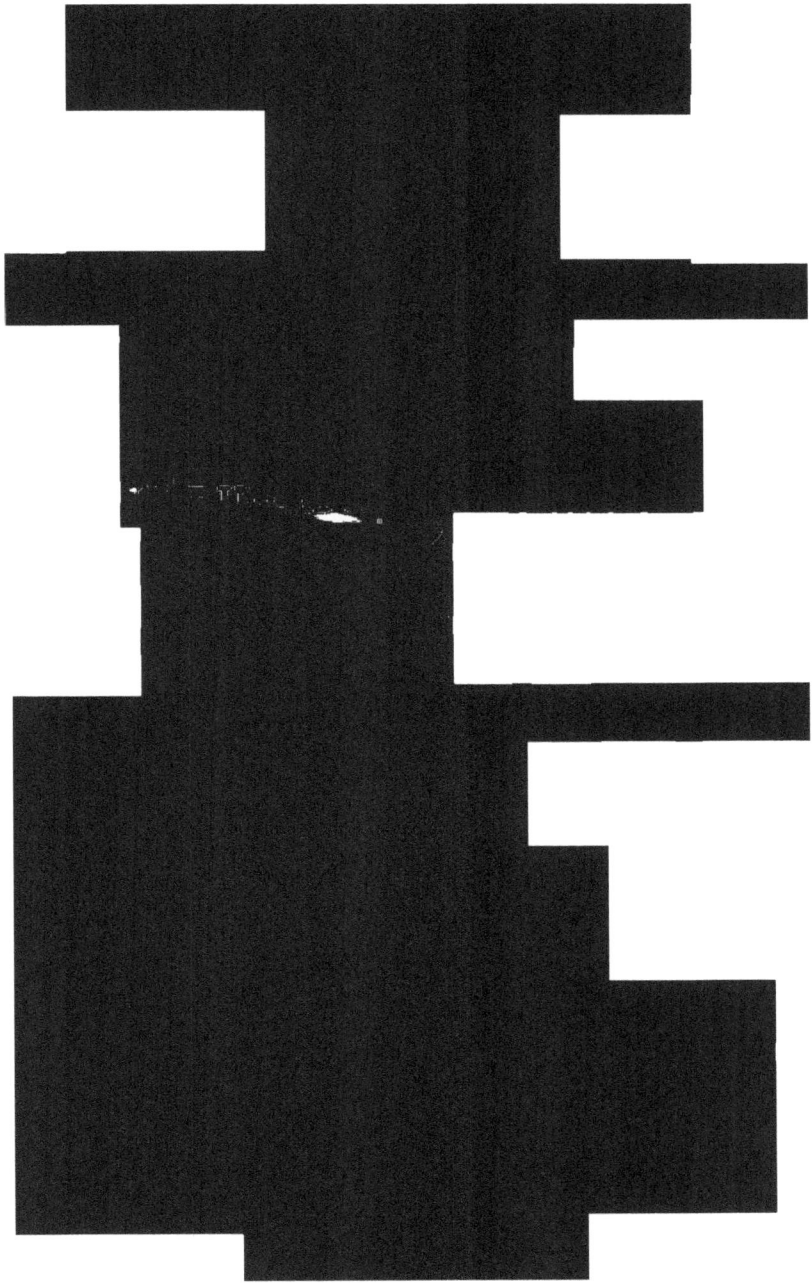

INTRODUCTION.

The study of disease, as a province of scientific knowledge, is called Pathology. It consists in the study of all morbid changes appreciable by the naked eye, or with the help of the microscope ; in the consideration of all anatomical changes, or lesions pertaining to disease ; in the enumerating of the great number and variety of phenomena or symptoms which disease gives rise to ; and closely connected with this, in the study of the means of discriminating, or diagnosis between the different diseases; a matter of great importance, both to the physician and to the patient

So far as I am aware, this is the only work treating of Sexual Pathology alone. The public have too long ignored as indelicate, or as unnecessary to be comprehended, except by those who are educated in all the branches of the medical profession, a knowledge of these matters ; these, if known, as are here presented, would be one of the most effectual means to prevent the increase of sensualism and licentiousness that now seems to have taken such a strong hold upon the youth in this age.

General ignorance prevails among all classes of society in regard to a subject which not only concerns the health and happiness of individuals, but the permanency even of the social fabric. Not until the unhappy victim struggles to escape the destruction that his sexual instincts have brought upon him is the knowledge found. It is a delicate task of imparting this information necessary to avert the calamity sure to follow indulgence. But it must be done, and whose better task is it, to raise his warning voice against those secret sins which sap the physical

and moral growth of the individual, to show up in all its hideous
colors the ills engendered by misguided passions, than the good
physician,—who makes a ministry of his art, who is the constant
spectator of human suffering. The dread of physical ills will
keep many of our youth from morbid desires and sensual indulgences and is a great incentive to virtuous habits. Terrible indeed
are the consequenses of licentiousness to the health of individuals,
and families, certain and dreadful is the retribution. Generations
yet to come are made the sufferers.

The evils are taught by one generation to that which follows,
and so general has this education of evil become that it is rare to
find those who have been fortunate to escape wholly from its
contamination. Unhappily the physical pollution is not all; the
mind becomes tainted. Associated with it are loose conversa-
tions, licentious imaginations, and low ideas of the relations of the
sexes. This leads to the reading of obscene, or at least voluptuous,
books, gazing upon pictures of the same description and to general licentiousness of thought and of language. When once the
mind becomes corrupted the pollution of the end can not be told.
Surely no one will say that we overstate the extent of this evil, or
exaggerate its importance to the health and morals of the young.

The object I have endeavored to attain in this small work is, to
present concise, yet thoroughly truthful and practical descriptions
of the principal diseases of the reproductive organs. I am pre-
paring, as the time from my professional duties will allow, and
will soon publish in connection the hygiene treatment and thera-
peutics of the diseases described in this work. It will comprise
about 300 pages.

As some time has elapsed since this work was first advertised
as in preparation and soon to be published, some apology for, or
explanation of the causes of the delay may be due to the public, and
more especially to those who have sent in their subscription and who
have awaited its appearance so patiently. The only reason why
its publication has been so long delayed was the want of time in
the engrossing duties of professional life.

While this treatise aims and claims to be, so far as anatomical and pathological problems are concerned, rigidly scientific, and to be posted, up to the time of going to press, in all the knowledge and facts of this rapidly advancing age, so far as they come within the scope of its plan and purpose, its style and arrangement are addressed to the populace rather than to the professional reader. Its sole object is to instruct the masses of the people on those subjects which have hitherto been to them as a sealed book.

In the first part of the work I have described the reproductive organs and the diseases Spermatorrhoea with Involuntary Emissions and Impotence and Sterility in male and female. In the second part I have described the Venereal diseases and their complications, also Nephrites, Lithiasis Prostatorrhoea, Prostatitis Diabetes.

These diseases are the great bane of the world. Hardly the person exists who does not know from experience or observation, their blighting effects. With the prudery which prevents the parent from cautioning his son, or the physician his patient, from these violations of every natural instinct and every physiological law, I have not the slightest patience.

Enfeebling to the body, enfeebling to the mind, the incarnation of selfishness, it effaces from its victim his fondness for the other sex, unfits him for true love, and likens him, in very fact, to that embodied concentration of all man's frailties, devoid of all the apparent virtues of animals, still lower in the scale, the ape.

This habit of self-abuse is resorted to from different motives. With many, there is no opportunity for the natural qualification of their appetites; some are deterred from such qualification by the fear of discovery, regard for character, or a dread of disease ; others there are whose consciences revolt at the idea of licentious intercourse, who yet addict themselves to this practice with the idea that there is in it less of criminality. It is to be apprehended, however, that its commencement can usually be traced to a period of life when no such causes can have been in operation. It is begun from imitation, and taught by example, long before the thoughts are likely to have been exercised, with regard either to its dangers or its criminality. The prevalence of this vice among boys there is great reason to believe, has very much to do with the great amount of illicit indulgence which exists among young men. The one bears the same relation to the other, in a certain sense, that moderate drinking does to intemperance. It prepares the way, it excites the appetite, it debauches the imagination. There is little doubt that it is often, if not commonly, begun at a period of life when the natural appetite does not, and should not exist. It is solicited, prematurely developed ; it is almost created. On every account, then, this practice in the young demands especial notice. It is the great corrupter of the morals of our youth, as well as a destroyer of their health and constitution. Could it be arrested, the task of preventing the more open form of licentiousness would be comparatively easy ; for it creates and establishes, at a very early age, a very strong physical propensity, an animal want of the most imperious nature, which, like the longing of the intemperate man, is almost beyond human power to overcome.

If the consideration of the matters here presented shall induce one to stay in his wild career, and to face about to a purer and better life I shall feel abundantly satisfied and well repaid for the labor.

C. BIGELOW.

277 & 279, S. Clark St., Chicago, Ill.

References have been made to the following works and authors : Acton's " Reproductive Organs" ; Durkee's "Venereal Diseases" ; Flint's "Practice of Medicine" ; Storer's " Is it I" ; Bartholow's "Spermatorrhoea" ; Walker's "Intermarriage" ; Ryan's " Philosophy of Marriage" ; Scudder's "Venereal Diseases" ; Trall's "Sexual Physiology" ; Hill's "Venereal Diseases" ; Rindfleisch's " Pathology".

SEXUAL PATHOLOGY.

PART FIRST.

THE SEXUAL ORGANS.

A brief description of the Anatomy of the Sexual Organs may refresh the mind of the reader, and give a better understanding of some of the subjects that are to be discussed.

In both sexes the sexual organs are alike surmounted by an eminence of cellular tissue enclosing fat, and covered with stout capilla or hairs. The integument receives an abundant supply of sensory nerves, which associate it with the organs of copulation. This elevation, called the *Mons Veneris* in the female, in some persons possesses sexual sense in a very high degree, and anything which excites it calls forth an increased circulation to and turgidity of the erectile tissue.

The sexual organs of both sexes may be divided into the external or copulative, and the internal or reproductive. The copulative organs are formed in part of erectile tissue, and are very abundantly supplied with nerves of sensation from the spinal cord and brain. The reproductive organs proper are principally supplied from the sympathetic nervous system.

IN THE MALE.

The organs of generation are the penis, the prostate gland, vesiculæ seminales, and the testes.

The penis is composed of two erectile bodies, the *corpora cavernosa,* and the *corpus spongiosum.* The first, or the corpus cavernosum, forms the upper or larger portion, and is the best example of an erectile tissue; it has an external fibrous membrane, or sheath, from the inner surface of which numerous fine lamellæ pass into the interior of the body, dividing its cavity into small compartments, which look like cells when they are inflated.

Within these is situated the plexus of veins upon which the peculiar erectile property of the organ mainly depends. It consists of short veins, which very closely interlace and anastomose with each other in all directions, and admit of great variation of size, collapsing in the passive state of the organ, but, for erection, capable of an amount of dilation, which exceeds beyond comparison that of the arteries and veins which convey the blood to and from them. The strong fibrous tissue lying in the intervals of the venus plexuses, and the outside fibrous membrane or sheath with which it is connected, limit the distension of the vessels, and, during the state of erection, give to the penis its condition of tension, and firmness. The second, or *corpus spongiosum,* forms the lower and smaller portion, and the extremity, or glans penis, and contains within it the canal of the urethra. The same general condition of vessels exists in this part, except around the urethra the fibrous tissue is much weaker than around the body of the penis, and around the glans there is none.

The penis has a very firm attachment to the bones of the pelvis, and is supported from above by a strong ligament. It is covered with a delicate integument, loosely attached to the body of the organ by fibrous tissue, and terminating in a fold—*the prepuce*—which has an attachment to the body of the organ behind the glans. The penis is, as seen, abundantly supplied with blood, and by the peculiar situation of a pair of muscles, the *erectores penis*, the veins are compressed, the organ made turgid with blood and thrown in a state of erection.

The glans penis is the principal point of reunion of the sensitive nerves of the virile organ, no other part which it regulates can be compared with it in this respect. In respect to richness in nerves, the glans penis yields to no other part of the economy, not even the organs of sense.

The male urethra extends from the neck of the bladder to the opening of the urethra. Its length in the adult is usually eight or nine inches; its course has a double curve in its flaccid state, but in the erect condition it forms only a single curve, the concavity of which is directed upwards. The widest and most dilatable part is that which passes through the prostate gland; here upon the floor of the canal is a little ridge of mucous membrane and its subjacent tissue, called the *Verumontanem*, or *Caput Gallinajinis*. When distended it serves to prevent the passage of the semen backward into the bladder. A depression on each side of this is perforated with numerous apertures, the *orifices of the ducts* from the *prostate gland*.

The *prostate gland* is a small glandular body surrounding the neck of the bladder and commencement of the urethra. In shape and size it very much resembles a horse-chestnut. Its secretion is a milky fluid, having an acid reaction, and presenting, on microscopic examination, molecular matter. This gland is frequently enlarged, and its ducts filled with concretions, especially in old age. It properly belongs to the sexual organs, furnishing a secretion to be admixed with that of the vesiculæ seminales and testicles.

Cowper's glands are two lobulated bodies of a yellowish color, about the size of peas, situated beneath the fore part of the membranous portion of the urethra, between the two layers of the deep fascia, and lying close behind the bulb. The excretory duct of each gland is nearly an inch in length, and passes obliquely forward beneath the mucous membrane, opening by a minute orifice on the floor of the urethra. Their function is not definitely known. They diminish in size in advanced age.

The *vesiculæ seminales* are situated between the base of the bladder and rectum. They are two lobulated membranous pouches, which probably serve as reservoirs of semen, though they furnish a secretion peculiar to themselves.

The *testes* are contained in a cutaneous pouch—the *scrotum,* which is divided into two lateral halves by a septum. They furnish the male sperm for the fertilization of the ovum, and discharge their secretion during copulation by ascending ducts, the *vasa deferentia,* which, passing upward through the inguinal rings, descend on the wall of the bladder to the vesiculæ seminales.

Lying upon the posterior border of each testis is a narrow, flattened body, termed the epididymis. Attached to the upper end of the epididymis is a small pedunculated body, the use of which is unknown.

IN THE FEMALE.

The external organs in the female are the *mons veneris,* already described, the *labia majora* and *minora,* the *clitoris,* the *meatus urinarius,* and the entrance of the *vagina,* the introitus to the reproductive organs proper.

The internal organs are the *uterus, Fallopian tubes* and *ovaries.* The *labia majora* are two more or less prominent cutaneous folds extending from the *mons veneris* to the perineum, containing areolar tissue, fat and erectile tissue. Their prominence depends, in most women, on the amount of adipose tissue, though in some the erectile tissue is in such proportion as to give prominence when the organs are excited.   Externally, the skin is covered with hair, and supplied with nerves from the same source as the *mons veneris*.   Within the fissure, the lining membrane gradually loses the character of the skin and assumes that of mucous membrane.

The *labia minora* are lesser folds of the lining mucous membrane, extending from the clitoris backward for three-fourths the extent of the opening. They contain a plexus of vessels, forming a species of erectile tissue, and vary very greatly in prominence and extent in different persons.

The *clitoris* is thought to be the analogue of the male penis, and to possess the sexual sense in greatest degree.   The truth is, probably, that it is a rudimentary organ, very like the male mammæ.   In some women it is large, and composed of erectile tissue; it is erected during vascular excitement, and being freely supplied with nerves, adds to the voluptousness of coition.   But in others it can scarcely be detected, even during excitation, though they possess the sexual sense as fully developed as the others.

The *meatus urinarius* is found immediately behind the clitoris, and from it may be traced the urethra, about an inch and a half in length, imbedded in the *vesico-vaginal* wall.   The urethra has an erectile coat, in some women remarkably developed, and it also is in a turgid condition during sexual excitement.

The *vagina* is a membranous canal, between five

and six inches in length along its posterior wall. It is composed of an external muscular coat, a middle layer of erectile tissue and an internal lining of mucous membrane. The muscular coat consists principally of longitudinal fibres, continuous with the superficial layer of the uterus. The amount of erectile tissue varies in different persons, and is most abundant at the lower part of the vagina. The mucous membrane shows an anterior and posterior ridge or *raphe*, and between them it is thrown into numerous transverse ridges or *rugæ*.

The mucous membrane of the vagina is reflected upon the dependant portion of the uterus—*the cervix uteri*—giving it an investment, and reflected in the os, being continuous with the mucous lining of the cavities of the uterus. In its entire extent it is abundantly supplied with nerves of sensation, but possesses the sexual sense in highest degree at its inferior and superior portions.

The *uterus* is a pyriform organ, resting upon and partly depending in the vagina. In the unimpregnated state it measures about three inches in length, two in breadth at its widest part, and an inch in thickness, and weighs from an ounce to an ounce and a half.

It is subdivided into *fundus, body* and *cervix*— the first being the superior portion above the Fallopian tubes, the second the portion between this and the neck, and the third the lower and constricted portion, principally dependent within the vagina,

The walls of the uterus are thick, the cavity being quite small, and are composed of three coats— an external of peritoneum investing the fundus and body, a middle coat of muscular tissue, which forms its chief bulk, and an internal lining of mucous membrane.

The muscular coat is composed of layers of fibres so arranged that there will be equal contraction upon the cavity from all directions toward the outlet. In the cervix their arrangement is such, that they can both open and close the os, and cause a vermicular movement from below upward. It has been thought that this muscular tissue was only called into action for the expulsion of the ovum, or some foreign body which, by its presence and growth, had aroused the development of the uterine muscular fibre. This, however, may be a mistake, for it is called into action during sexual excitement, and is active during the venereal organism.

The circulation of the uterus is peculiar, and closely resembles erectile tissue in the tortuous course of the vessels, their free *anastomosis* and direct communication of many arteries and veins without the intervention of capillaries. The increased vascularity of the organ during the excitement of ovulation has long been noticed, and also that a similar state is produced by sexual excitement, though not to the same degree.

The *Fallopian tubes* lead from the uterus to the

ovaries, and are the conduits for the ova. Each tube is about four inches in length, and is terminated by an expansion—the *fimbriated* extremity—which is applied to the ovary during ovulation.

The *ovaries* are to the female what the testes are to the male, furnishing the germ of the future being. The ovary shows some fifteen or twenty ova in various stages of development, though in the tissue may be seen the germs of many others. They are discharged at each menstrual period, from puberty until it ceases at the "change of life." The nerves are principally from the sympathetic system, though a branch from the uterine system (sexual) passes upward and along the Fallopian tubes.

NORMAL FUNCTIONS OF THE REPRODUCTIVE ORGANS.

In youth and childhood sexual impressions should never effect a child's mind or body. All its vital energy should be employed in constructing the growing frame, in storing up external impressions, and in educating the brain to receive them. During a well-regulated childhood, and in the case of ordinary temperaments, there is no temptation to infringe this primary law of nature. The sexes, it is true, are allowed unrestricted companionship. Experience shows, however, that this intimacy is, in the main, unattended with evil results. In the immense majority of instances, indeed, it is of great benefit. At a very early age the pastimes of the girl and boy diverge; the boy takes to more

boisterous amusements, and affects the society of
boys older than himself, simply because they make
rougher, or, in his opinion, manlier playfellows;
the quieter games of girls are despised, and their
society is to a considerable extent deserted. This
apparent rudeness, often lamented over by anxious
parents, may almost be regarded as a provision of
nature against possible danger. At any rate, in
healthy subjects, and especially in children brought
up in the pure air and amid the simple amusements
of the country, perfect freedom from, and, indeed,
total ignorance of any sexual affection is, as it
should always be, the rule. The first and only feeling exhibited between the sexes in the young
should be that pure fraternal and sisterly affection
which it is the glory of our home life to create and
foster, with all its softening influences on the after
life. Education, of course, still further separates
children as they grow into boys and girls; and the
instinctive and powerful check of natural modesty
is an additional safeguard. Thus it happens that
with most healthy and well brought up children, no
sexual notion or feeling has ever entered their
heads, even in the way of speculation. I believe
that such children's curiosity is seldom excited on
these subjects, except as the results of suggestions
by persons older than themselves.

Puberty is distinguished by the advance in the
evolution of the generative apparatus in both sexes,
and by the acquirement of its power of functional

activity. At this epoch a considerable change takes place in the bodily constitution; the sexual organs undergo a much increased development, various parts of the surfaces, in the male, especially, the chin and the pubes, become covered with hair; the larynx enlarges and the voice becomes lower in pitch, as well as rougher and more powerful, and new feelings and desires are awakened in the mind. To the use of the sexual organs for the continuance of his race man is prompted by a powerful instinctive desire, which he shares with the lower animals. This instinct, like the other propensities, is excited by sensations; and these may either originate in the sexual organs themselves, or may be excited through the organs of special sense. Thus, in man it is most powerfully aroused by impressions conveyed through the sight or touch, but in many other animals the auditory and olfactory organs communicate impressions which have an equal power, and it is not improbable that in certain morbidly excited states of feeling, the same may be the case with ourselves.

Now commences the season of completed manhood—virility. Puberty is a season of change and preparation. The constitution is summoning all its powers to prepare the individual properly to protect and provide for his own wants, and to transmit life to future generations. Virility is the term of growth completed, of bones hardened, of vague and fleeting fancies of youth transformed into well-defined yearnings for home and children and a help-meet. Then is it right for the male to exercise those functions peculiarly his own; and then, only when this is accomplished as a subordinate act, conformed to moral and social law, and accessory to pure mental emotions. At the outset of his career he should learn by heart that in proportion as the human being makes the temporary gratification of the mere sexual appetite his chief object, and overlooks the happiness arising from spiritual communion, which is not only purer, but more permanent, and of which a renewal may be anticipated in another world—does he degrade himself to a level with the brutes that perish. But the distinctive sign of completed manhood is in the character of the secretion, which now commences. The secretion peculiar to the male, known as the seed or sperm, depends for its life-transmitting power on the presence of certain minute vibratory bodies, about one-fortieth of a line in length, called spermatozoa. These are exceedingly numerous and active when the secretion is healthy. A single one of them—and there are many hundreds in a drop—is sufficient to bring about conception in the female. They have a rapid vibratory motion, and great vitality. They are not, however, always present, and when present, may be of variable activity. In young men just past puberty and in aged men they are often scarce and languid in motion. Occasionally they are entirely absent in otherwise hale men, and this is one of the causes of sterility in the male. Their presence or absence can only be detected by the microscope. The organs in which this secretion is elaborated from the blood are the testicles. Previous to birth these small, rounded, firm bodies are in the abdomen, and only descend a short time before the child is born. They are composed of a vast number of minute tubes, united together by connective tissue. The total length of the tubes is estimated at forty-eight hundred feet, or nearly one mile. Nevertheless, so small are they that their full capacity is not more than six cubic *centimetres*

The left testicle, though usually suspended lower than the right, is somewhat smaller, the difference in weight being about ten grains. The secretion is most active about twenty-five years of age, and decreases after this period as age advances. It is, however, not constant, depending very much on physical and moral causes. In some men it is periodical or intermittent, and they are therefore entirely impotent at times, without at all impairing their vigor at other times.

The testicles are subject to special diseases, which may seriously impair their action. Mumps sometimes changes from the face to them, causing painful swelling; and frequently a similar attack occurs in venereal diseases. Inflammation may arise from an injury, and also from violent and ungratified sexual excitement. All these affections may lead to loss of power, and sterility, and it does not answer, therefore, to neglect them.

Diseases which are not connected with the genital organs do not seem to produce any after influence on the secretion in the adult in middle life, but in aged persons, on the other hand, this is a frequent occurrence. From the moment that the evolution of the generative organs commences (the testicles act), if the texture is not accidentally destroyed, they will continue to secrete up to a very advanced age. It is true that the secretion may be diminished by the absence of all excitement, direct or indirect, by the momentary feebleness of the economy, or by the action of special medicines ; but it never entirely ceases from puberty up to old age.

And now begins the trial which every healthy youth must encounter, and from which he may come out victorious, if he is to be all that he can and ought to be. The child should know nothing of this trial, and ought never to be disturbed with one sexual feeling or thought. But with puberty a very different state of things arises. A new *power* is present to be exercised, a new *want* to be satisfied. It is, I take it, of vital importance that boys and young men should know, not only the *guilt* of an illicit indulgence of their dawning passions, but also the *danger* of straining an immature power, and the solemn truth that the *want* will be an irresistible tyrant only to those who have lent it strength by yielding; that the only true safety lies in keeping even the thoughts pure. Nothing, I feel convinced, but a frank statement of the truth will persuade those entering on puberty that these new feelings, power and delights, must not be indulged.

The instinct of reproduction, when once aroused, even though very obscurely felt, acts in man upon his mental faculties and moral feelings, and thus becomes the source, though almost unconsciously so to the individual, of the tendency to form that kind of attachment towards one of the opposite sex, which is known as *love.* This tendency, except in men who have degraded themselves to the level of brutes, is not merely an appetite or emotion, since it is the result of the combined operations of the reason, the imagination, the moral feelings and the physical desire. It is just in this connection of the physical attachment with the more corporeal instinct, that the difference between the sexual relations of man and those of the lower animals lies. " Nuptial love maketh mankind, friendly love perfecteth it, but wanton love corrupteth and debaseth it." Here, then, is the problem. A natural instinct, a great longing, has arisen in a boy's heart, together with the appearance of the powers requisite to gratify it. Everything—the habits of the world, the keen appetite of youth for all that is new—the example of companions—the pride of health and strength—opportunity—all combine to urge him to give the rein to what seems a natural

propensity. Such indulgence is, indeed, not natural, for man is not a mere animal, and the nobler
parts of his nature cry out against the violation of
their sanctity. Nay, more : such indulgence is
fatal. It may be repented of. Some of its consequences may be recovered from ; but from Solo-
mon's time to ours, it is true that it leads to a
" house of death."

PROPHYLAXIS.

Every man who is wise must feel that no help
is to be despised in any part of the life-battle all
have to fight. And in that struggle for purity,
which is at least for the young the hardest part
of it, what help to seek and where and how to
seek it, are no unimportant questions, and in a
practical treatise well deserve a few words.

One of the most important aids to youth in
preserving a pure and healthy mind, as also a pure
and healthy body, is that power of the mind over
outer circumstances which we call a *strong will.*
Without this resolute grasp of the intellect and
and moral nature to direct, control and thoroughly
master all the animal instincts, a man's life is but
an aimless, rudderless drifting, at the mercy of
every gust of passion or breeze of inclination towards tolerably certain shipwreck.

This command of the man over himself and his
outward circumstances is a matter of habit. Every
victory strengthens him, until, after years of cour-

ageous self-rule, it seems impossible for him even to yield.

This steady discipline of the will has a direct physical effect on the body. The steady avoidance of all impure thoughts—the turning away, so to speak, of the will from sexual subjects—will take away much of the distress and temptation arising from the abnormal excitement of the body and reproductive system.

The essence of all this training of the will, however, lies in beginning *early*. If a boy is once impressed fully that all such indulgences are dirty and mean, and with the whole force of his unimpaired energy, determines he will not disgrace himself by yielding, a very bright and happy future is before him.

It is not, however, sufficient to train and strengthen the mind and will; the body must be subjected to a regular and determined discipline before the proper command can be obtained over its rebellious instincts. And this discipline will not consist in any violation of the natural rules of health, but in a strict conformity to the hygienic regulations which science has proved must be obeyed before real health and vigor can be ensured.

Abstinence from fermented drinks and exciting animal food, avoidance of over-eating and moderation in diet, and an active hygiene exercise and gymnastics are most essential and worthy of all trial.

SPERMATORRHŒA, OR NERVOUS DEBILITY.

This is an effect rather than a cause—a *symptom* rather than a *disease.* It means the effect of an *unnatural discharge of the semen* or *seminal fluid.*

Sometimes profuse, often but slight, but always involuntary; hence the difficulty is sometimes called Involuntary Emissions. These generally occur at night, and usually during sleep; but sometimes, in bad cases, in day time, and both day and night.

There is a close and constant sympathy existing between all the various organs of the human system; so that if one organ or class of organs suffers, the others do, and the whole system partakes of the suffering. This is often and easily noticed in case the stomach or bowels are diseased or out of order. A diseased or disordered stomach gives a sick headache; a diarrhea soon weakens and prostrates the whole system; if the liver is out of order, the whole body soon feels the consequence. But it may truly be said, that the sympathy which exists between the Generative Organs and the balance of the system is stronger and more intimate than that of any other class of organs. Hence, when the generative system is deranged, debilitated and out of order, the whole organization, physical and mental, body and mind, soon becomes also deranged and out of order—the whole system soon feels the effect. How must it be, then, when this deranged and diseased condition of the generative system is kept up and continued? The generative organs are the source of life; they lie at the very foundation of life; their derangement, therefore, if continued long, must soon derange the whole system, mind as well as body; for that balance which maintains health is destroyed; functional derangement supersedes harmonious action—the body loses its vitality, its energy; it is no longer properly nutrified and cannot be; chronic derangement spreads throughout the system; disease of body and of mind becomes fixed, and the unhappy victim drags out a miserable life or sinks into an untimely grave.

Of all the diseases or derangements which affect or which can affect the generative organs, there is none equal nor half so bad as *Spermatorrhœa.* All others together, or one after another, in a continuous round, are not capable of producing—and never have and never can produce—half so much mischief, derangement and ruined health, as this one evil of Spermatorrhœa or involuntary emission of Semen! It is a direct draft upon the vital energies of life itself, destroying both body and mind as it goes! And the longer it continues, the more difficult it becomes to overcome. This fact, of course, must be apparent to every one.

INVOLUNTARY EMISSIONS or Spermatorrhœa, may be and is produced by various causes, though by far the most common and prolific cause is that which is called Onanism, Masturbation or Self-Abuse, of which I shall speak more fully presently. In some instances, it is a constitutional weakness, independent of all controlling circumstances or known causes—inherent in the person. In other words, it is congenital, and has been inherited as the effect of ancestral vices or defects in constitution. In such cases it is more difficult to cure. It has also been known to follow injuries to the brain, or to that portion of the brain called the *cerebellum*, which is the lower and back part of the brain. It still more commonly results, however, from disease of the *prostate gland*, which may be produced by various causes—among which are excessive venereal or sexual indulgencies; by neglected or improperly treated Gonorrhea, and by Self-Abuse. It may also result from general or great debility of the whole system. But by far the most common cause is that vicious and secret habit of self-pollution. There need hardly be anything said as to the symptoms of Spermatorrhœa or Involuntary Emissions. The disease is as I have said—an involuntary discharge of a fluid from the genital organ, called the Semen. It is the same as that which is discharged or emitted in the act of coition or sexual intercourse. This involuntary emission takes place generally, or most commonly, at night, while the patient or subject is asleep. He dreams, for instance, of some lascivious matter, and while thus dreaming the genital organ becomes excited, the same or similarly as when in the act of coition, and there is a discharge of semen, or of some fluid resembling semen. It may be partly semen and partly some other secretion. This may be repeated, so that there may be several such emissions during the night. And by-and-by, as the habit increases and the weakness becomes worse, these emissions become more frequent, and will occur whenever the victim sleeps, whether he dream or not. And finally it increases to such an extent that it will occur during the day, on the least sexual excitement of the organ. As a matter of course, it becomes not only a great annoyance to the unhappy victim, but is a constant draft upon his vital powers and energies, undermining and sapping the very foundation of his life, destroying his energies, both of body and mind, and making him shun society and become disgusted with himself and the world around him.

Says a French author, who has written extensively on this subject :

"These patients soon become ill; their most intimate friends are ignorant of the cause of the various disorders they complain of ; the medical man who possesses their confidence is not better informed, for even the patients themselves entertain no suspicions of the real nature of their complaint. Hence their disposition is to settle down into ennui, tendency to melancholy, or to hypochondriasis. When their disease assumes a more serious aspect, then the constitution is said to be delicate, impressionable, or unhealthy, and they are looked upon as *malades imaginaires*. They are reproached with too much care of themselves, or an overfondness for medicine. Medical men in extensive practice tire of hearing the tale of so long a series of unintelligible and inexplicable maladies, and rid themselves of such patients by recommending them to travel, or a change of air. Charlatans plunder them; officious friends advise marriage, or some sort of occupation to fill up the void in their existence ; but all blame them, because none really comprehend the nature of their disorder. Unfit for any serious occupation, and incapable of deep reflection, they become dissatisfied with themselves and still more so with others. Absorbed in one sole thought, they return incessantly to themselves to seek for the cause of their lamentable condition, and soon become misanthropical."

This applies very well—indeed describes exactly, one class of the victims to this lamentable disorder—those in high life or easy circumstances, persons of leisure, and especially *females.* It is but a mild description, mildly drawn, and of but a small number compared with the thousands that suffer from the same cause. There are thousands whose cases and conditions are much worse than would be supposed from the above description, and who know also *what ails them,* but nevertheless will not tell their physician, or make known to him or to their best friends even, the true state of their case. They know the cause of their trouble, and know also that it is carrying them down to ruin; yet they cling to it, either believing that nothing can save

them—that there is no remedy—or else prefer inevitable ruin to the exposure of their case and their
horrid vice to a physician. Such is the enchanting
power of this evil over its victim, when it once gets
entire control over him.

But still there are other thousands who do not
really know what it is that ails them, or rather what
has caused, and perhaps is still causing, their unhappy condition. They have never been properly
informed on the subject. Their parents, either
from a false delicacy or from ignorance, have failed
to properly instruct them when young, of the dangers which lay in their path, and warn them
against them; and they have never, perhaps, read
of their danger in any book that has fallen into
their hands. How, then, should they know?

Next to the parents, I hold it to be the *duty* of
the *physician* to see to it that the youth of our land
shall be properly instructed on this subject, and
where parents feel such a delicacy that they cannot
or will not do it, they ought to have their family
physician perform the duty. But above all, whoever writes a book like this, on the subject of secret
diseases and vices, should by all means speak fully
and plainly on this greatest, the most debasing, the
most common, and the most terrible and ruinous
in its effects, of all the vices and evils of the age,
and of all ages. It is the curse of manhood, and
destroyer of the race. All other evils and vices to
which the human race is addicted, or subject, are

but as the drop in the bucket in comparison with this evil and the VICE which is its prolific CAUSE.

CAUSES OF SPERMATORRHŒA.

This distressing and debilitating condition is induced by various causes, though in a vast majority of cases it originates from one common cause, or secret vice.   And in order to treat a case properly and successfully, it will always be necessary to know the cause, and if possible, *remove* it.   Remove the cause is the proper way to cure nearly all complaints.   It is especially important in this disease.

As to the different causes of Spermatorrhœa, I shall now speak of but one—the main, or common cause.

One of the strongest passions or desires to which man is subject is that of *sexual feeling.*   The God of Nature has implanted this desire or feeling in mankind for one of the wisest and most important purposes—that of propagating the species, and for causing that proper feeling to exist between the two sexes which is absolutely necessary, and which could not exist, were it not for this propensity.   Next to the desire for food, there is probably no desire to which animated nature—animals as well as men— is subject, that is so strong and imperative as this known as the sexual desire. To *live* and to *give life* are the dominant passions.   Yet this sexual desire is not so much that of giving or imparting life, as it is a desire to *enjoy the pleasurable feeling of the act.* Hence it leads the young, who have arrived at that age when this desire becomes fully developed—the age of *puberty,* as it is called—to make use of other means than the natural and legitimate one to incite and produce that pleasurable emotion or feeling which is caused by the sexual act, or act of coition.

All creatures seem to have their pro-creative desire. Providence, as I have said, has rendered this so, in order that they may propagate their species. Beasts, birds, reptiles, insects and all the lower order of animals below that of man, it would seem, have a stated and fixed period or season of the year, for sexual commerce or intercourse, and are never found violating this law of nature. Of all created and creating animals, man appears to be the only one that allows his sexual passions and appetites to run counter to the wise provisions and regulations of nature in this respect. And hence, man being the only transgressor of the law in this matter, is the only animal or being that suffers such a thing as disease of the sexual organs, such as are described in this book. But man alone, of all created beings in this world, is furnished with reasoning powers; the knowledge of good and evil is set before him, or given to him, and he knows, or ought to know, that he must *control* his feelings, and keep them within bounds; and when he fails to do so, it is but right and proper that he suffer the penalty.

At puberty, perhaps, or about the time the youth verges into manhood, as I have said before, the sexual propensity is stronger, or the desire greater than at any other time. But it is very evident that this propensity, though it may be ever so strong, ought not to be indulged freely at this period. Sexual indulgence at this early period of life is always attended with more or less evil consequences to the heedless and misguided youth. Manhood should be in full vigor and maturity before sexual intercourse should be indulged in. To propagate the species, the progenitors should be perfect and in a full state of perfection, otherwise, the act can but be injurious to those who indulge in it, and the fruits of the act must lack that degree of perfection which is desirable, and which parents in the full development of manhood and womanhood are capable of producing. But if sexual intercourse at too young an age, or before the young man is fully developed and matured, is injurious, how much more injurious is that dreadful vice called onanism, masturbation, or self-pollution.

This vice is sometimes due to a disease. Thus it can be occasioned by an eczema of the genital parts, by errors of conformation (*phymosis, paraphymosis*), by the accumulation of the sebaceous matter, the existence of worms in the rectum, leucorrhœa, priapism, nymphomania, diseases of the cerebellum, idiocy, pulmonary phthisis. It has been remarked that certain positions while awake and during sleep, conditions which require the person to be ordinarily seated, (tailors, shoemakers, dressmakers, seamstresses,) the administration of purgatives, above all, of aloes, the use of aphrodisiac substances, fish species, alcoholic liquors, especially beer, favor the development of masturbation. However, masturbation is more frequently caused by the premature excitement of the genital organs, by precocious desires, provoked by a disorderly imagination, brought on by an enervating and sensual education. It is, above all, in boarding-schools that the contagion of bad example exercises its fatal ravages. Sometimes it is to early childhood that we must go back to find the first cause of disgraceful and ruinous habits. Domestics, as stupid as corrupt, masters, who ought to be the guardians of innocence, do not recoil before the infamy of making beings without reason subserve their odious lubricity.

The word *masturbation* is from the two original words — *manus* — hand, and *stupro* — to commit adultery. It means, in plain terms, to excite the genital organ by titilation with the hand, so as to produce that peculiar and thrilling sensation which is experienced in the natural and healthy act of coition, or sexual intercourse between the sexes. The word *Onanism* is derived, it is said, from Onan, spoken of in the Bible, as a man who was guilty of this horrid practice. But it matters little what the names given to this vice are derived from, or what they originally meant: it is the vice itself with which we have to do, and every body knows what it is, and what is meant, for almost every body is, or has been at some time of his or her life, guilty of the practice, to a greater or less extent. It is to-day the prevailing and great degenerating vice of the race! or of the young, of all classes, conditions, and of both sexes! yes, of both sexes, for girls and young women are guilty of it, as well as young men and boys—though, it is hoped and believed, to a much less extent than the male sex. My own experience, at least, will corroborate the fact that it exists to a much less extent among females than it does among males. Nevertheless, it is a lamentable fact that the habit, or vice, as it should be called, exists among both sexes, and among all classes of society, and all ages. The church, even, is not exempt from it. It is an unnatural and unlawful use of the organs which were given by the Creator to mankind for wise and beneficent purposes—for the continuance and reproduction of the human race—in accordance with the divine injunction, as proclaimed to man at the Creation, and recorded in the first chapter of Genesis—in the memorable words: " Be fruitful and multiply, and replenish the earth."

It is a disgraceful fact, that this vice can be traced back to the remotest periods of antiquity, and that it has been practised by the highest as well as the lowest classes of society, in all ages and countries from that time to the present. But it is believed that at no period of the world did the vice prevail to such an alarming extent, and so generally through society, as at the present time. To such an extent is the sin practiced, that comparatively few of our youth are free from it. Our boarding-schools, common schools and colleges are full of it; while adults, as well as the young, indulge in it to an extent that would be shocking to the public sense, were it publicly known.

The effects of this vice are much worse upon the young than upon the adult and middle aged; it is a lamentable fact that it is often known among children, who are initiated into the practice by nurses and servants. How important, therefore, is it that something should be done to put a stop to, or, at least, to check this terrible and demoralizing vice. So deadly is the infatuation of this vice to a young man, that the first indulgence by which he enters the path of the onanist might also claim the lines which Dante has inscribed over the gate of hell:

> " Through me you pass into the city of woe,
> · Through me you pass into eternal pain,
> Through me, among the people lost for aye.
> * * * * * *
> All hope abandon ye who enter here."

Parents, teachers, guardians, ministers, physicians and moralists everywhere should, in some way or other, portray to the rising generation the baneful effect of this secret, solitary vice, for there can be no doubt that at this very moment it is doing more injury to bodily health, mental vigor, and purity of morals, than all other evils and vices put together. Physiologists agree that the loss of *one ounce of semen* is more debilitating than the loss of *forty ounces* of blood. Hippocrates supposed that the male semen was composed of all the fluids of the body, and considered it the most precious constituent of the human organism. Pythagoras terms the semen the flower of the blood. Others of the ancient physicians considered the semen a portion of the brain, and Epicurus even looked upon it as a mixture of soul and body. But one thing we all know; by losing semen we lose vital energy or principle, and it is not to be wondered at, therefore, that the excessive loss of semen should enervate and destroy body and mind.

But the loss of semen is not the sole cause (as is generally supposed) of sexual debility. This is proved by the nervous depression coming on in young children from sexual excitement before they can be said to secrete semen. Similar exhausting nervous effects are noticed in women who do not secrete any such fluid, but merely mucous; and yet many experience the nervous orgasm or spasm, which acts as harmfully on them, when much indulged in, as on males. This spent secretion contains no spermatozoa. What passes, if examined under the microscope, consists of mucous, or the debris of epithelium. Nevertheless, as an effect of long-continued and often repeated shocks, women become subject to epileptiform attacks, and various nervous affections, as well as local affections of the uterus, direct consequences of masturbation. The womb, as has been well observed, is the centre around which women's sentient feelings radiate. No one who has treated a large number of women laboring under uterine affections, but must have been struck with the haggard, feverish, pinched cast of countenance, which too often characteristically denotes the existence of long-standing uterine affections. The immediate cause of this nervous depression has, within the last few years, excited a good deal of attention; and the conclusion has come that there is a good deal of evidence now existing which shows that shocks constantly received and frequently repeated on the great nervous centres, produce irritation in them, and thus causes many of the obscure forms of disease, to which there has hitherto been no key. And when these nervous centres are irritated, the spinal chord also becomes irritated and diseased, so that undue excitement of the generative functions may set up irritation of these nervous centres, and this undue excitement will be communicated to the spinal chord, producing depression of spirits, pain at the pit of the stomach, and general prostration. An able writer thus speaks of the morbid state of the nervous system induced by excesses:

"The morbid state of the nervous system—more particularly of the spinal chord—which is produced by masturbation, is analogous to that which is observed in muscles after excessive exercise. The history of some of the cases of progressive muscular wasting away makes it evident that in some persons the excessive employment of single muscles, or groups of muscles, may lead to their complete wasting away; and that this atrophy may be manifested in different ways. In the natural exercise of a muscle its composition and texture are, in however small a measure, changed; fatigue is the sensation, we have of the changed state of the muscle, or its nerves; and the state is one of impairment, for the muscle has lost power. In health, and the natural course of events, the repair of the thus impaired muscle is accomplished during the repose which follows exercise. But if due repose be not allowed, the impairments may accumulate, and the muscles may become gradually weaker, so as to need greater stimulus for the fulfillment of their ordinary work; and at length, in some instances, they may even lose the power of repairing themselves during repose. Now, although the very nature and products of the changes that ensue in nervous organs during their exercise are less well known than are those that ensue in muscles, yet the occurrence of such change is certain. And it seems a fair analogy which suggests that the loss of nervous power that follows long-continued *masturbation* are due to changes parallel with those that are witnessed in the progressive muscular wasting away after excessive muscular exercise—the softening and wasting of the

spinal chord being essentially similar to that traced
in muscles. It is taken for granted here, that the
act of masturbation is associated with what may be
regarded as violent exercise of the spinal chord."

So, we see, besides the loss of semen in itself,
· the repeated shocks given by this fearful habit to
the nervous centres have a great deal to do in
producing this loss of nervous power.

It has been urged in excuse or palliation for this
vice of masturbation, by those who indulged in it—
especially members of the church—that their sexual
passions were so strong they could not control
them; that they must have vent of some kind, and
that they resorted to this secret habit to prevent or
save them from committing fornication! But this
is a most disgraceful as well as false excuse. One
might as well urge in palliation for theft that his
desire to steal was so strong he could not control it,
and to keep from stealing other people's goods he
took to stealing his own! The parallel will be perfect if we substitute *destroy* for the word *steal*, for
whoever indulges in this secret vice *destroys his
own health*, of body and mind, more certainly and
lamentably than by any other vice or habit he could
indulge in. Besides, it is not true that the sexual
passion is too strong to be controlled, or that it must
be indulged, in some way or other. There is no
man nor woman whose constitution is ordinarily
perfect, or who is of ordinary mind, but can control
this passion and keep it subdued, if they try. Let

them but control their evil and lascivious thoughts
and imaginations.   There lies the secret of the whole
matter.   It is not true that *continence*, or abstaining
from sexual indulgence, is detrimental to health.   I
know it has often been argued that it is; and many,
a deluded victim has been encouraged to practice
this vice or continue it, on account of such belief—
the belief that if he did not give vent to his pent-
up sexual energies, his health would become injured, or he would lose all sexual desire and power!
Never was there a greater or more fatal delusion.
I admit that, at a proper age—say from twenty-five
to thirty years—it would be better, and more in accordance with nature, for all healthy persons to
marry.   But perfect celibacy or abstinence forever
from sexual indulgence is a thousand times better
than even the most moderate indulgence in this
secret vice of which I have been speaking—this
self-pollution and self-destruction of body, soul and
mind!   A life of celibacy is never the cause of *impotence* nor of *sterility*.   It is the *abuse* of the sexual organs that causes both of these conditions,
more frequently than all other causes put together
—abuse just in this way, by *masturbation* or *onanism*.   But impotency and sterility are but of trifling
consequence in comparison with the other frightful
consequences which often result from this horrid
vice.   It destroys the whole nervous system, or deranges it to the extent of producing various nervous
disorders, and many other serious complaints which

go to make up a catalogue of the most frightful diseases to which flesh is heir. Consumption, heart disease (functional), insanity are the most common results of this evil. It is safe to say that at least two-thirds of all the nervous diseases are caused by this single vice! But who can measure the evil or calculate the suffering caused by it, simply in the form of *bad health*, without any particular name or disease? It is a *disease* itself, with innumerable unpleasant and distressing *symptoms*, and tends directly to impair and finally destroy the entire nervous system; leading to ruined health, imbecility, idiocy and insanity! But as I have undertaken to go into this matter thoroughly, and to lay it bare before the reader and the world, so that all who read this exposure may be informed thoroughly and be without excuse, I must now enter into more detail. Before going any further, however, let me repeat that the semen is the most concentrated and most precious fluid or secretion of the human body. Its production is slow in the continent man—so slowly that, in fact, in many instances, I think little or none is formed in healthy adults whose attention is not directed to sexual objects, and who take a great deal of strong exercise.

The semen, however, as emitted, is not the semen as it is secreted in the testes. It may be said, while in the testicles, to be in little more than a rudimentary state. When ejaculated, it is a highly **elaborated** secretion.

None, iu fact, amongst the various secretions of
the body seems to require so much time to mature.
Not only have cells to be formed and thrown off,
as in the case of other secretions, but after they are
liberated in the testicles, they have to divide and
multiply, and each division to become, through a
gradual growth, an adult Spermatozoon. When
thus prepared, it is passed down the spermatic chords
to the reservoirs, *vesiculae seminales;* there it is
mixed with the secretion of the prostate gland,
and also with that of the vesiculæ. This dilution
seems to render it more fluid, and thus more capable of passing easily along its course. It has
been stated by a celebrated English anatomist
(Monro), that if the little—almost imperceptible—
ducts or *canals* through which this secretion is
carried to its general receptacle were united in one,
they would reach over *five thousand feet!* With
all this apparatus, and delicate and complex preparation, no wonder then that this fluid is precious,
and that its waste and the derangement of its
secretion cause disastrous consequence to the
whole system, but especially to that of the nervous.
Spermatorrhea, as I have said, is an involuntary
discharge of this precious fluid—the semen. The
common and almost universal cause of this disease
—Spermatorrhœa—is self-abuse of the genital organs in the manner already described. This habit or
practice of self-abuse generally commences when
the victim is quite young—long before puberty,

or the full growth of the person. When it is continued until puberty and afterward, it is almost sure to lead to Nervous Debility, or an involuntary discharge of the Semen, which will take place at night, when the victim is asleep—often several times during the night. And if it continues— that is, if nothing is done to cure it, and the patient also continues the habit of self-abuse, this involuntary discharge of Semen will occur also during day time; and it may become so bad that the Semen will be constantly passing off, in the urine, as well as at other times.

Now let us draw a brief picture of a victim to this secret vice of self-abuse or self-pollution, known as Onanism or Masturbation. We take the youth —a boy of perhaps twelve or fourteen years—though it is often commenced at a much earlier age—one boy teaching the habit to another or others, younger than himself, and perhaps also at school—for it is well known that our schools are the very hot- beds of this vice, among both sexes.

The boy has acquired the vice. It produces a new and pleasing—a rapturous-sensation. He has no idea that it will hurt him. He likes it. In- dulgence in it soon becomes a daily practice. And soon, not only daily, but several times a day. Watch him, and you will soon find that he steals away, several times a day, or is absent—somewhere by himself! Ten chances to one it is to indulge in this secret vice! Not only, however, during

the day will it be indulged in.   At night, also, on
retiring to bed, and in the morning again on
waking and before getting up, will it be done.
And not unfrequently, on waking during the night,
perhaps with lascivious dreams, will the victim
indulge in this now confirmed habit.   You will
find the sheets stained, or his linen, with the wasted
Semen!   How often, alas! do parents see and know
this, and yet say nothing to their children!

The effect of the habit soon becomes visible to
all around.   They may not know what is the trouble or the cause, but they can see easily enough
that something is the matter with the boy.   He
loses his bright, ruddy and healthy complexion;
his face becomes pale with, most likely, a bluish
tint around the eyes, which are sunken and have
lost their luster.   The lips lose their deep red
color and look pale.   The mind also is affected.
The subject will sit, perhaps, as if engaged in deep
thought, without looking at anything.   He becomes
averse to play and to the society of others, and
loves to be alone.   He is disposed to sleep late of
a morning, but without being refreshed on getting
up; complains of weariness, heaviness, and pains
in the limbs and back.   The appetite becomes impaired and various; indigestion is imperfect; the
tongue covered with a thick, whitish coat; the
whole face and appearance looks emaciated; the
mind wanders, the intellect becomes weaker instead
of stronger, and it is now evident to parents and

all who see him that something serious is the
matter. Yet who knows or who will say what it
is? Who will tell the boy, now verging almost
into manhood, it may be—who will tell him what
it is that is ruining him, and will snatch him from
inevitable destruction, before it is too late? Very
likely the father knows, or strongly suspects, what
it is that ails his boy, but lacks the courage or
the resolution to tell him. But where is the "family physician?" Does he not see this boy, and
does he not know that he is in the downward road
to ruin? Why does he not do his duty? for I
hold that it is the duty of every true physician,
as a conservator of the public health, as the minister of the Gospel is that of the public morals, to
see to just such cases as these; and especially is
it the duty of the "family physician"—by which I
mean simply, the physician who is in the habit of
attending that family. Where parents cannot make
up their minds to give their children—especially
their boys—the proper instructions on this subject,
they ought by all means to place the matter in the
hands of some good physician, whose experience
and influence will help to carry conviction home
to the young sinner, and who may thus be saved
from a horrid life or more horrid death, by timely
reformation. How often is it, however, that the
young life is allowed to perish for want of proper
and timely instruction, even before it has begun

to bud, as a young plant withers away, at whose root a worm has been gnawing?

But that so important a matter as this is may not be left with the reader to rest entirely upon my word and what I may say, I will now copy the following, which is translated from the writings of one of the most distinguished and learned physicians and physiologists of Germany. Here is what he says in regard to *Spermatorrhœa* and that Secret Vice which is its prolific cause:

"Hideous and frightful is the stamp which Nature fixes on one guilty of unnatural excesses. He is a faded rose—a tree without a bud—a *wandering corse!* All life and fire are killed by this *secret cause*, and nothing is left but weakness, inactivity, deadly paleness, wasting of body, and depression of mind. The eye loses its luster and strength; the eye-ball sinks; the features become lengthened; the fair appearance of youth departs, and the face acquires a pale, yellow, leaden tint. The whole body becomes sickly and morbidly sensitive; the muscular power is lost; sleep brings no refreshment; every movement becomes disagreeable; the feet refuse to carry the body; the hands tremble; pains are felt in all the limbs: the senses lose their power, and all gayety is destroyed. Boys who before showed wit and genius, sink into mediocrity, and even become blockheads; the mind loses its taste for all good and lofty ideas, and the imagination is utterly vitiated. Every glance at a female form excites desire. Anxiety, repentance, shame and despair of any remedy for the evil, make the painful state of such a young man complete. His whole life is a series of secret reproaches, distressing feelings, self-deserved weakness, indecision, and weariness of life; and it is no wonder if the *inclination to suicide* ultimately arises—an inclination to which none is so prone as those who are, or have been, given to *self-abuse.* The dreadful experience of a *living* death renders *actual* death a desirable consummation. The waste of that which *gives* life (the semen) generally produces disgust and weariness of life, and leads to that peculiar kind of destruction which is characteristic of our age. Moreover, the digestive power is destroyed; flatulence and pains in the stomach are likely to follow, and create constant annoyance; the blood is vitiated; the chest is obstructed; eruptions and pimples break out upon the skin; the whole body becomes dried and wasted; and in the end comes slow fever, fainting fits, epilepsy, palsy, consumption, insanity, and an early death!"

This is the brief and summary statement of but one out of many that I might produce, of men of the greatest eminence and reliability.

A distinguished professor of France, noted for his skill and experience in these matters, thus remarks concerning the commencement of this vice:

" However young the children may be, they get thin, pale, and irritable, and their features become

haggard.   We notice the sunken eye; the long, ca-
daverous-looking countenance; the downcast look,
which seems to arise from a consciousness in the
boy that his habits are suspected, and at a later period, from the ascertained fact that his virility is
lost.   I wish by no means to assert that every boy
unable to look another in the face is, or has been, a
Masturbator, but I believe this vice is a very frequent cause of timidity.   Habitual masturbators
have a dank, moist, cold hand, very characteristic
of great vital exhaustion; their sleep is short, and
most complete atrophy comes on; they may gradually waste away if the evil passion is not got the
be:ter of; nervous symptoms set in, such as spasmodic contraction, or partial or entire convulsive
movements, together with epilepsy, and a species of
paralysis accompanied with contractions of the
limbs."

It is no more horrible than true, as may be exemplified in thousands of cases all around us to-day.
Look around you and see if you cannot pick out
just such cases among your own acquaintances.
You will see just such cases.   You may not know
what ails them.   They may not even themselves
know what is the cause of their troubles.   But
could the truth be ascertained, ten chances to one,
their case and its cause has been described and accounted for in the above sketch.

Of course all cases are not so bad as the above.
But thousands of cases are worse.   This is not a

medium picture. All will become as bad as this, if continued; and while the unhappy victim gives himself up entirely to unnatural beastiality and lustful desire of this kind, he will ultimately find himself in a condition worse even than is here described.

Speaking of the sin and the dreadful consequences of masturbation or self-pollution, Dr. Adam Clarke says: "The sin of self-pollution is one of the most destructive evils ever practiced by fallen man; in many respects it is several degrees worse than common whoredom, and has in its train more awful consequences. It excites the powers of nature to undue action, and produces violent secretions, which necessarily and speedily exhausts the vital principle and energy; hence the muscles become flaccid and feeble—the tone and natural action of the nerves relaxed and impeded; the understanding confused; the memory oblivious; the judgment perverted; the will indeterminate, and wholly without energy to resist. The eyes appear languishing and without expression, and the countenance becomes vacant; appetite ceases, as the stomach is incapable of performing its proper office, and nutrition fails; tremors, fears and terrors are generated. And thus the wretched victim drags out a miserable existence, till superannuated even before he had time to arrive at man's estate, with a mind often debilitated, even to a state of idiotism, his worthless body tumbles into the grave and his guilty soul is hurried into the awful presence of its Judge!"

How truly and well does the great Commentator describe the effects of this besetting evil of our race. It is true as Holy Writ, and ought to be inscribed in every school book in the land, or placed where the young and rising generation could read it every day.

But here is a Report, which is so important and so much to the point, that I could hardly think I had done justice to this subject, if I should omit copying a large portion of it. It is a Report on the subject of *Idiocy*, presented to the Legislature of the State of Massachusetts, in February, 1848, by *Dr. Howe*, in obedience to a resolution of that body, directing a Report to be made on this appalling subject. Says that Report :

" There is another vice, a monster so hideous in mien, so disgusting in feature, altogether so beastly and loathsome, that in very shame and cowardice, it hides its head by day, and vampyre-like, sucks the very life-blood from its victims by night; and it may, perhaps, commit more direct ravages upon the strength and reason of those victims than even intemperance; and that is, SELF-ABUSE.

"One would fain be spared the sickening task of dealing with this disgusting subject; but, as he who would exterminate the wild beasts that ravage his fields, must not fear to enter their dark and noisome dens, and drag them out of their lair—so he who would rid humanity of a pest, must not shrink from dragging it from its hiding-place, to perish in the light of day. If men deified him who delivered Lerna from its hydra, and canonized him who rid Ireland of its serpents, what should they do for one who would extirpate this monster vice? What is the ravage of fields, the slaughter of flocks, or even the poison of serpents, compared with that pollution of body and soul, that utter extinction of reason, and that degradation of beings made in God's image, to a condition which it would be an insult to the animals to call beastly, and which is so often the consequence of excessive indulgence in this vice.

" It cannot be that such loathsome wrecks of humanity as men and women, reduced to drivelling idiocy by this cause, should be permitted to float upon the tide of life without some useful purpose; and the only one we can conceive, is that of awful beacons to make others avoid—as they would moral pollution and death—the cause which leads to such ruin. This may seem to be extravagant language, but there can be no exaggeration, for there can be no adequate description even of the horrible condition to which men and women are reduced by this horrible practice. There are, among those enumerated in this Report, some who not long ago were considered young gentlemen and ladies, but who are now moping idiots—idiots of the lowest kind; lost to all reason, to all moral sense, to all shame; idiots who have but one thought, one wish, one passion; and

that is, the further indulgence in the habit which
has already loosed the silver cord in their early
youth; which has already wasted, and, as it were,
dissolved the fibrous part of their bodies, and utterly extinguished their minds.

"In such extreme cases, there is nothing left to
appeal to—absolutely less than there is in dogs or
horses, for they may be acted upon by fear of pun-
ishment—but these poor creatures are beyond all
fear and all hope, and they cumber the earth awhile
—living masses of corruption. If only such lost
and helpless wretches existed, it would be a duty to
cover them charitably with the veil of concealment,
and hide them from the public eye, as things too
hideous to be seen; but, alas! they are only the
most unfortunate members of a large class. They
have sunk down into the abyss towards which
thousands are tending! The vice which has shorn
these poor creatures of the fairest attributes of humanity, is acting upon others, in a less degree,
indeed, but still most injuriously—enervating the
body, weakening the mind, and polluting the soul.
A knowledge of the extent to which this one vice
prevails would astonish and shock many. It is,
indeed, a pestilence which walketh in darkness,
because, while it saps and weakens all the higher
qualities of the mind, it so strengthens low cunning
and deceit, that the victim goes on in his habit
unsuspected, until he is arrested by some one whose
practiced eye reads his sin in the very means which

he takes to conceal it—or until all sense of shame is forever lost in the night of idiocy, with which his day closes.

" Many a child who confides everything else to a loving parent, conceals this practice in its innermost heart. The sons and daughters who dutifully, conscientiously and religiously, confess themselves to father, mother, or priest, on every other subject, never allude to this. Nay, they strive to cheat and deceive by false appearances: for, as against this darling sin, duty, conscience and religion are all nothing. They even think to cheat God, or cheat themselves into the belief that He who is of purer eyes than to behold iniquity, can still regard their sin with favor.

" Many a fond parent looks with wondering anxiety upon the puny frame, the feeble purpose, the fitful humors of a dear child, and, after trying all other remedies to restore him to vigor of body and vigor of mind, goes journeying about from place to place, hoping to leave the offending cause behind, while the victim hugs the disgusting serpent closely to his bosom, and conceals it carefully in his vestment!

" The evils which this sinful habit work, in a direct and positive manner, are not so appreciable, perhaps, as that which it effects in an indirect and negative way. For one victim which it leads down to the depths of idiocy, there are scores and hundreds whom it makes *shame-faced, languid, irreso-*

lute, and inefficient for any high purpose of life. In this way the evils to individuals and to the country is very great.

"It behooves every parent — especially those whose children (of either sex) are obliged to live and sleep with other children—whether in boarding-schools, boarding-houses, or elsewhere, to have a constant and watchful eye over them, with a special view to this pernicious and insidious habit. The symptoms of it are easily learned. Nothing is more false than the common doctrine of delicacy and reserve in the treatment of this habit. All *hints,* all *indirect* advice, all attempts to cure it by creating *diversions,* will generally do nothing but *increase* the *cunning* with which it is concealed. The only way is to *throw aside all reserve;* to charge the offence directly home; to show up its disgusting nature and hideous consequences in glowing colors; to apply the cautery seething hot, and press it into the very quick, unsparingly and unceasingly.

"Much good may be done by the publication of cheap books upon this subject. They should be put into the hands of all youth suspected of the vice. They should be forced to attend to the subject. There should be no squeamishness about it. There need be no fear of weakening virtue, by letting it look upon such hideous deformity as this vice presents. Virtue is not salt, or sugar, to be softened by such exposure, but the crystal or diamond that repels all foulness from its surface. Acquaintance with such a vice as this—such acquaintance, that is, as is gained by having it held up before the eyes in all its ugliness—can only serve to make it detested and avoided.

"Were this the place to show the utter fallacy of the notion that harm is done by talking or writing to the young about this vice, it could, perhaps, be done by argument—certainly by the relation of a pretty extensive experience. This experience has shown that in ninety-nine cases in a hundred, the existence of the vice was known to the young, but not known in its true deformity; and that in the hundredth, the repulsive character in which it was first presented made it certain that no further acquaintance with it would be sought. There are cases recorded where servant women who had charge of little girls, deliberately taught them the habits of self-abuse, in order that they might exhaust themselves and go to sleep quietly. This has happened in private houses, as well as in alms-houses; and such little girls *have become idiotic!* The mind instinctively recoils from giving credit to such atrocious guilt; nevertheless, it is there, with all its hideous consequences; and no hiding of our eyes, no wearing of rose-colored spectacles—nothing but looking at it in its naked deformity, will ever enable men to cure it. The above remarks forcibly apply to all our public schools, for I have become too well acquainted, I was about to say, with the alarming extent to which it prevails, often in the most open manner. The extent of it is amazing, for it exists both among the teachers and the students, and what can be more absurd than the partial, even, shunning of the subject? By so doing, it leads, not only to the continuance in some, but the production of it in the yet uninitiated. From this may be inferred that it is a pest, generally engendered by too intimate association of persons of the same sex; that it is handed from one to another, like contagion, and that those who are not exposed to the contagion are not likely to contract the dreadful habit. Hence, we see that not only propriety and decency, but motives of prudence require us to train up all children to habits of modesty and reserve. Children, as they approach adolescence, (or puberty,) should never be permitted to sleep together. Indeed, the rule should be—not with a view only to preventing this vice, but in view of many other considerations—that after the infant has left its mother's arms and becomes a child, it should ever after sleep in a bed by itself. The older children grow and the nearer they approach to youth, the more important does this become. Boys even should be taught to shrink sensitively from any unnecessary exposure of the person before each other; they should be trained to habits of delicacy and self-respect; and the capacity which nature has given to all for becoming truly modest and refined, should be cultivated to the utmost. Habits of self-respect, delicacy and refinement, with regard to the person, are powerful adjuncts to moral virtues. They need not be confined to the wealthy and favored classes; they cost nothing—on the contrary,they are the seeds which may be had without price, but which ripen into fruits of enjoyment that no money can buy."

The foregoing is but one out of many authorities of the most solemn and grave character, which might be quoted from in condemnation of this destructive and much deprecated vice, and in evidence of the alarming extent to which it prevails. COPELAND, in a work on Insanity, in which he points out its various causes, sets this horrid vice down as one of the most prolific causes of insanity, and holds the following language in regard to it:

"Many, however, of those causes which thus affect nervous energy, favor congestion of the brain and occasion disease of the genital organs, tending to disorder the functions of the brain sympathetically. Of these, the most influential are Masturbation and Libertinism, or sexual excesses—sensuality in all its forms, and inordinate indulgence in the use of intoxicating substances and stimulants. The baneful influence of the first of these causes—self-abuse, or Masturbation—is very much greater, in both sexes, than is usually supposed, and is, I believe, a growing evil, with the diffusion of luxury, of precocious knowledge, and of the vices of civilization. It is even more prevalent in the female than in the male sex, and in the former it usually occasions various disorders connected with the sexual organs—as leucorrhœa—suppressed or profuse men-struation—both regular and irregular hysteria—catalepsy, ecstacies, vertigo, and various states of disordered sensibility, before it gives rise to mental disorder. Melancholia, the several grades of dementia, especially imbecility and monomania, are the more frequent forms of derangement proceeding from a vice which not only prostrates the physical powers, but also impairs the intellect, debases the moral affections, and altogether degrades the individual in the scale of social existence, even when manifest insanity does not arise from it."

An ordinary result of spermatorrhœa is weakness of mind. The brain acts slowly and imperfectly, because a larger part of the produced nerve force is consumed in the frequently repeated venereal orgasm. These patients are dull and listless. To accomplish a given amount of intellectual labor, they find that an unusual effort is necessary. They are given to reverie, and to vague and shadowy dreams, in which erratic phantasms play. They take little interest in business and in the affairs of life; and to this cause is to be attributed, in many instances, unexpected failure in business and professional pursuits. They are men of dreams instead of men of ideas and action. There is diminished sensibility. The respiration becomes more or less irregular. Frequent deep inspirations, sighing and a dry cough are often observed. Dryness of the fauces, and huskiness of voice also occur. Irregular action of the heart is most common. Pains are felt in this region, the rhythm of the heart's movement is altered, and a subjective sense of fluttering is felt. These phenomena are frequently accompanied by a sense of constriction of the throat—a *globus hyster-icus*—a tendency to shed tears, and the emission of a plentiful quantity of pale urine. Amongst the serious results are impotence, irritable testes, varicocele and insanity.

The Massachusetts report says that one hundred and ninety-one of the idiots examined were known to have practiced Masturbation, and in nineteen of them the habit was even countenanced by the parents or nurses! One hundred and sixteen of this number were males, and seventy-five were females. In four hundred and twenty who were born idiots, one hundred and two were addicted to *Masturbation*, and in ten cases the idiocy of the children was manifestly attributable to self-abuse in the parents. The ten cases known justify the conclusion that in reality there are many more, which proves, beyond a shadow of a doubt, that many cases of idiocy in children are attributable to the sexual vice of the parents. Is not this fact almost too fearful for contemplation, and the importance of it to the community incalculable? A number of the ablest and best men of the medical profession have written upon this subject at different periods during the last twenty years, and some long before, and all in the most pointed and unqualified condemnation of the habit as among the most ruinous of vices.

In an able treatise of insanity in young men, a celebrated physician thus describes the symptoms premonitory and general:

" The parent, after her son (the only child, it may be) is taken to an asylum, will tell you that his insanity cannot be accounted for. He has been so well conducted, so quiet and studious, not seeking the company of the gay, the idle and the thoughtless, but remaining quietly at home rather than joining the social amusements of those of his own age. Further inquiry may elicit that he has been of good abilities, and, it may be, clever in his occupation; that he had few friends, and rather shunned the society of those of the other sex. Had he been other than he was, some cause might have been found in the irregularities of life to cause insanity in one scarcely beyond boyhood's years; but in such a quiet lad, and so carefully brought up, she is unable to suppose a cause. Then she may tell you that for some time past a gradual alteration has been going on; he has changed, not only in manner, but in appearance; he has become so peevish and irritable, so reserved in his conversation, so apathetic in manner, so slovenly in dress, so contradictory and so uncertain in his actions, so hesitating, first determining on one thing, and before he could execute that, changing to some other course, and has shown such a want of self-reliance. That quite recently he has grown more

and more apathetic, more slovenly in dress, paying
less attention to cleanliness, and becoming slower in
his actions; that he is now not only irritable in his
temper, but is, at times, violent; that he does things
by 'fits and starts,' is impulsive, deliberating long
and then suddenly hastens, apparently, to carry out
his intention; and has become so stupid-looking
and lost, and incapable of taking care either of
himself or his business; and all this has occurred
without any apparent cause, except it may be his
studious habits. At last, he can be borne with no
longer; he is unmanageable in a private house, and
is obliged to be removed from his home." And so
we notice one particular class of symptoms, that of
apathy, irritability of temper, want of self-reliance,
uncleanly and slovenly in dress; quiet, and wishing
to be alone, and shunning the society of the opposite sex, in those under the influence of this vice,
whose minds are turning.

On entering an asylum for the insane, especially
if it be one receiving patients from the middle as
well as from the lower class of society, there is one
group of inmates which may arrest the attention of
the visitor, from the contrast presented to the excited persons around him on the one hand, and to
those who are convalescent on the other. Engaged
in no social diversion, the patients of this group
live alone in the midst of many. In their exercise,
they choose the quietest and most unfrequented
parts of the airing-grounds. They join in no social

conversation, nor enter with others into any amusement. They walk alone or they sit alone. If engaged in reading, they talk not to others of what they may have read ; their desire apparently is, in the midst of numbers to be in solitude. They seek no social joys, nor is the wish for fellowship evinced. The pale complexion, the emaciated form, the slouching gait, the clammy palm, the glassy or leaden eye, and the averted gaze, indicate the lunatic victim to this vice.

Apathy, loss of memory, abeyance of concentrative power and weakness of mind generally, combined with loss of self-reliance, and an indisposition for any kind of action, irritability of temper, and incoherence of language, are the most characteristic mental phenomena of chronic dementia, resulting from masturbation in young men. As in diseases of an exhaustive nature, we find that the cutaneous secretion is poured forth abundantly, so in the cases occupying our attention, the perspiration breaks forth on the slightest exertion. This relaxed condition of the perspiratory system is especially marked in the palms, and the exception is to find these dry in the masturbator; for, generally, a damp, or cold, clammy perspiration is always present, and makes it particularly disagreeable to take the hand of one of these persons. The gait is slovenly or slouching, and the gaze is downcast or averted; and, when addressed, the masturbator does not look the speaker openly in the face whilst he replies, but looks to the ground or beyond the questioner. The physical system is, as a rule, but indifferently developed. The muscles are small, soft and flabby; the body is generally emaciated, the adipose tissue being but feebly stored up; the complexion is variable, but though occasionally flushed, is, as a rule, pale.

How many persons have been the victims of their lustful passions! Medical men, every day, meet with those who, by this means, are rendered idiotic, or so enervated, both in body and in mind, that they drag out a miserable existence; others perish with marasmus (wasting away of the flesh), and too many die of a real pulmonary consumption. Mr. Woodbridge, in the "Annals of Education," says: "This fatal vice is spreading desolation throughout our schools and families, unnoticed and unknown. Our boarding schools and day schools are sources of untold mischief."

You may examine every boy you meet, from ten to eighteen years of age, and, could the truth be ascertained, one out of every ten will be found addicted to the habit, at least. At any rate, this will be found to be true with all who have arrived at the age of puberty—fully this many are given to the polluting and destroying vice.

Mrs. Gove, in her "Lectures to Ladies on Anatomy and Physiology," says: "About twenty years since, my mind was awakened to examine this subject, by the perusal of a medical work that described the effects of this vice when practiced by females. This was the first intimation I had that the vice existed among our sex. Since that time I have had much evidence that it is fearfully common among them. There is reason to believe, that in nine cases out of ten, those unhappy females who are tenants of houses of ill-fame have been victims of this vice in the first place. Professed Christians are among its victims."

Indeed, it may be said that there is enough written and published on this subject, if it were of the right kind, and in a shape suitable for the class intended. Nearly every medical work that is written of late has more or less to say about it, and in condemnation of the evil. But, unfortunately, these books are not read by the victims of the habit—not being intended for such readers, nor adapted to their capacity. What is wanted are small-books and tracts, written in a style to be understood, and which shall press home the matter to the understanding and comprehension of the humblest reader, and that will be felt and heeded even by the most depraved victim, if his reason is not yet entirely gone, nor shame forsook his breast.

Venereal diseases have done much, and are doing much to disease, weaken and demoralize the physical constitution of the human family—even in some parts of the world to the extent of depopulating the country (as in the Pacific Islands); but they are as but the drop in the bucket compared

with this great vice. Insanity, idiocy, and imbecility of mind are some of its fruitful effects;
while impaired health, ruined constitutions, diseases of various kinds, impotency and general debility are its certain effects upon the body. It is
an evil which cries aloud for a remedy, and appeals
to every parent, every guardian of the young—to
the moralist, the humanitarian, the physician, the
minister of religion, and to the teacher, to aid in
counteracting its effects and its progress. The only
remedy is to *break it up* entirely!—to stop it!
Through a mistaken and false idea of *morality*,
and *delicacy* and *modesty*, this vice has been winked
at, or suffered to pass unrebuked by parents, cler-
gymen and physicians. It is time all such false
notions of delicacy and modesty were thrown aside.
What are modesty and morality worth if they
allow children and the youth of our land to go to
ruin? No false delicacy should ever be suffered to
stand between a father and the welfare and health
of his son, nor between mother and daughter.

The criminal habit of solitary Onanism or Masturbation is the most pernicious kind of debauchery, on account of its frightful results. In my
opinion, neither pestilence, nor war, nor variola,
nor a host of similar ills, has results more disastrous
for humanity. It is the destructive element of
civilized societies; and it is much the more active,
inasmuch as it acts constantly and ruins population
little by little. On this point there exists a unanimous

accord amongst all physicians. And let it not be
supposed that physicians wish to exaggerate the
dangers attributed to solitary pleasures. They do
not. Of all venereal excesses, masturbation presents the most dangerous. Let us see why. A
great number of circumstances render difficult or
prevent intercourse with women; but this impu-
dicity never finds any obstacle. So, also, it has no
bounds; as soon as it has subjugated the heart, it
holds an odious empire over the senses; everywhere
it pursues, without cessation it harasses, provoking
lascivious ideas and desires, even in the midst of
most serious occupations. Hence results the so frequent repetition of its acts.

The mind and the body concur in soliciting to
evil. The imagination, beset by immodest thoughts,
excites to unruly acts. The genital organs, excited
by the morbid activity of the function, secrete the
prolific fluid more abundantly, and require more
and more often to be relieved. The habit becomes
then so powerful, that it enchains its victim and
reigns despotically, holding him under the yoke of
servitude, and, as the will becomes progressively
enervated, as well as the body, there comes a time
when the unfortunate one, feeling the cruel restraints of the evil, wishes to correct himself, but is
unable; he has neither sufficient force nor courage.
" I have within me two desires," said a young man
to me, endowed with the finest qualities of mind,
but who used himself up in consequence of his

passion, "one which resists and the other which leads me on. This latter, in order to seduce me, makes use of the most adroit subterfuge, and always says to me, 'This will be the last time.'" The unfortunate young man died of pulmonary disease. To the sufferings which weigh down the body are added the pains which torture the soul.

In the pleasures of love, the heart partakes of the enjoyment of the senses; and this joy, by favoring digestion, by animating the circulation, by provoking all of the functions, to a certain extent, to repairs the losses of the organism. But in Onanism, in this odious theft made against nature, in this strange perturbation of the genital sense, there is found nothing but regrets, sadness, shame, and remorse. The crime is so infamous, even in the eyes of him who commits it, that he will never dare to acknowledge his licentiousness, and that he will envelope himself in the shadows of mystery in order to give himself up to his fornication. How many even have perished from never having dared to declare the cause of their ills? "We could excuse him," says a writer, "who, seduced by a desire that nature has imprinted in the heart, and which he makes use of for the propagation of the species, has only done wrong in abusing it, and injuring himself. But for him, unfortunate one, he sins against all laws, he corrupts all the sentiments, he deranges the most admirable designs of the Creator."

So it seems to him that every one reads upon
his countenance the cause of his degradation.
You see him shun society, forsake pleasures, plunge
himself in the most profound isolation, a prey to
a sombre melancholy, tormented by the remorse
of having been himself the artificer of his own
physical and moral ruin; he cannot sometimes
even more aspire to the sweet consolation of marriage; he does not, and he can not, for all women
are to him a horror.

One of the most common results of Spermatorrhœa is *Impotency;* that is, inability to perform the
act of sexual intercourse, and to beget a child.   In
partial impotency, the patient may be able to perform the act, however, and yet not be able to become a father.   But if the disease is allowed to
continue, it is certain to result in complete impotency.   Hence, no one with Spermatorrhœa, even
but in a mild form, should think of matrimony or
of marrying a wife, until first being cured of it
and restored to entire health and soundness of
the genital organs.   I have treated, within
the last ten years, a large number of cases of this
distressing complaint.   Indeed, I have made its
study and treatment a *specialty*, to a certain extent, for a number of years past, and think I know
something of its character, its treatment, and the
alarming extent to which it prevails.   Impotency
is vastly more common than any one not familiar
with the matter would ever suppose.   At least a

certain degree of impotency, as for instance, where the person, though he may be able to beget a child, yet cannot more than half perform the act or enjoy its pleasurable emotions. In nine cases out of every ten, of such persons, this partial impotency has been caused by self-abuse before marriage.

But there is relief for such unfortunates. They can be cured, if they do not put off the matter too long. I have cured a large number of cases of complete impotency, or of what appeared to be such—where the patient was utterly unable to perform the act of coition at all. While in cases of but partial impotency, I never think of failing to effect a cure. To all persons, therefore, and to young men especially, who contemplate matrimony at some time or other, and who are troubled in this way at all, whether little or much, whether partial or complete, I would say—and I say it candidly and honestly—apply to a physician—to a skillful physician —to one who knows what to do, who understands the difficulty and knows how to relieve it. I do not say apply to me. It may be impossible or very difficult for you to do that. But my advice is— apply to some one in whom you have confidence, and good reason to believe that he is honest, skillful, and able to relieve you.

But Impotency is not by any means the only bad effect of Spermatorrhœa. When once established, it is one of the most distressing and life-destroying complaints that can affect the human body.

It is the gradual and constant wasting of one of the most precious and highly concentrated fluids or secretions of the body. Spermatorrhœa, once fully established, not only consists in nocturnal emissions, or involuntary discharges of the semen when the victim is asleep, but this discharge takes place at other times and in various other ways, often unknown or unperceived by the patient. It often becomes so bad that the semen passes off with the urine when the patient makes water, and also when at stool. And all this may occur without the patient being aware of it; and if he is aware of it he may not know half the extent to which it occurs, nor be aware of half the danger under which he labors. Such is the insidious nature of the disease.

I have already alluded to the condition of Spermatorrhœa—called "Nocturnal" or Nightly "Emissions"—but refer to it again, because it is the most common form under which the complaint occurs. There are thousands of persons, both male and female, who are subject to nightly emissions of semen, but who never say anything about the matter or make any effort to have themselves cured of it, until the disease has assumed a more serious form, and for the double reason that they do not know what ails them, and do not think it is a matter of any consequence, or that it *can* be cured. And thus they let it run on, perhaps for years, until it has become a serious and confirmed case of Spermatorrhœa,—the emissions occuring both day and night, on the least sexual excitement of the organs, and until perhaps the semen begins to pass off when at urine and at stool as stated.

These nightly emissions, as well as all forms of Spermatorrhœa, are of course much more common among young men and males, than among females, as is the deplorable habit of self-abuse. And it is much more injurious to males than to females. Impotency, occasioned by Masturbation and Spermatorrhœa, is ten times more common among males than among females. And my object in recurring to this form of the disease again—to Nocturnal Emissions—is to call the special attention of young men to the subject, and to endeavor to impress upon them the danger to which they are liable, if they have become, even in the least, subject to these emissions, and the importance of their taking measures at once to be relieved. For if the matter is neglected and the difficulty is allowed to run on, it will surely become worse, and will eventually lead to confirmed Spermatorrhœa and Impotency. These Nocturnal Emissions occur usually when the patient is asleep, and, as I have already said, by the patient dreaming of sexual intercourse or excitement, which causes an erection of the sexual organ. And finally, the disease and its cause act mutually on each other—each increasing the other. In other words, lascivious dreams cause erections, and emissions tend to encourage such dreams; and thus it is easy to see how natural and certain it is for the patient, once having . become subject to nightly emissions, to grow worse, or for the weakness to increase. Whoever, therefore, finds that he is, even but in the smallest degree, subject to emissions of this kind, or is even troubled with nightly erections of the penis—for this latter will lead to emissions—should seek advice and assistance from some good physician, and that without delay. It will be very easy, comparatively speaking, to cure the disease in this early stage, or even when these nightly emissions have become regular and well developed. The worst cases of simple "nocturnal emissions" are easily cured, compared with confirmed Spermatorrhœa, Nervous Debility and Impotency, and where the emissions occur day and night. In short, the sooner the disease is taken in hand and properly treated, the easier will it be to cure, or to restore the patient to health and vigor; while, on the other hand, the longer this is delayed or put off, the more difficult will it be to effect a complete cure. Hence my advice is—and I am conscious that I give it disinterestedly and from the purest of motives—whenever you discover that there is anything wrong with your genital organs—no matter what—where you even suspect or fear that such is the case—go direct to a physician, and to the best one you can find or know of for that kind of practice. If he is an honest man, as he should be, he will tell what

is the matter, if anything, and also what to do or have
done. There are hundreds of men who would give
a princely fortune to be rid of this single disease of
Spermatorrhœa, in some of its many forms, and be
perfectly sound and healthy in their genital organs.
There are hundreds of young men in our country
now subject to at least " nightly emissions," who
are blindly, unthoughtedly, tending rapidly to this
same condition, which, if they do not attend to the
matter in time, will certainly by-and-by reach it,
when they, too, would give all they were worth, and
ten times more, if they could be restored to health
and soundness in those organs. And there are
thousands more, of our youth—young men and
women—who are in the downward road of ruined
health—who are daily practicing the ruinous vice
of Masturbation and Self-Pollution, who, if not
saved in time, will make shipwreck of their health,
both of body and mind, and of all their hopes and
the hopes of their friends. If this book falls into
the hands of any such—and we know it will, into
the hands of *many* such—we say to them, as the
last and most important advice we can give, and as
we would to our own son—Beware of this deadly
vice—this bane of human happiness and earthly
hopes! Beware! Abstain! Break it off—or you
are surely ruined ! If you cannot save yourself
from this dreadful enemy—call to your aid the advice and assistance of a skillful physician; put your

case in his hands; do as he tells you, and you may yet be saved.

MATRIMONIAL CHASTITY.

The union of man and woman has not alone for its end the rekindling without cessation of the flame of life; it ought still more to associate together souls, to put in common the diverse faculties of each being, to complete one by the other, and to contribute in that way to their happiness and their moral perfection. Thus it is necessary that love should partake more of the soul than of the body. Sensual love, so transitory, so monotonous, ought to be controlled and purified by the love of the heart, so durable, so varied; one should be made subordinate to the other. Then we shall have modesty and chastity there. Moral love, not dependent alone on the passionate senses of youth, but attaching itself to the soul, can alone remain, and remains, faithful, because the soul alone can remain always beautiful.

Truly, man ought to know well all the evils with which he is threatened by the abuse of sensual pleasures. He ought to know what these mistakes of a disordered passion, these intoxications with immoderate lust, must cost for his soul, for his body, for his health, for the duration of his life, for his progeny. If so many men do not attain their whole physical and moral destinies, if they do not raise themselves to the highest intellectual conceptions, if they are burdened by diseases, if they see death decimate the race, if they do not arrive at the term of longevity marked out by nature, they can often blame themselves; for they themselves have been the artificers of their premature ruin.

They have hastened to gather, in their flower, all the pleasures of life. They have contaminated and squandered in advance the enjoyments reserved for mature age. They have exhausted themselves, with an insensate furor, in enervating sensual pleasures, which consume the resources of the organization and the vital forces. Then, have glutted themselves before their time; they are, also, before their time, enfeebled, decrepit, *impotent*, and, when they think to procreate a family, they have only left to them the remnants of a languishing life, which can only produce a bloated race. You see, in the great cities, these beings whom debauchery has blighted. They are wasted, pale, stunted in physique; in morals they vegetate in idleness, egotists, senseless, incapable of resisting evil, capable of all the vices.

We must raise our voice against the dangerous abuses which soil the conjugal bed, against onanism of man and wife. We do not enter upon this subject without regret; but this vice is so widely spread that science should take cognizance of it. It should make known the real dangers of these artificial relations, invented by a culpable fraud, to prevent fecundation, and to annihilate the natural

consequences of thé conjugal relations. It is painful
to avow how much, in our age, this vice is propa-
gated; and how much it propagates itself still,
from day to day, in all classes of society. It seems
in this respect, as if the moral sense were lost, a
condition of things which permits of disorder without any scruple. There, then, assuredly, is a shameful social wound. How, then, has it come to us?
Fatal maxims have been scattered in society. In
the name of a false science, it has been maintained
that populations cannot continue to increase, because the alimentary substances do not increase in
the same proportions; that it is necessary, consequently, to restrain generation, to limit the family,
to hinder, above all, or retard the marriages of poor
persons, in order not to arrive at a dearth, and not
to augment pauperism. On the other hand, luxury
increasing more and more beyond the limits of for-
tunes, individuals looking too much to the future
have wished to limit their progeny to their
resources, in order not to divide up their revenues
too much, and scatter their riches. Let us add to
these causes the weakening of religious beliefs and
practices. Religion, whose moral prescriptions are
in perfect harmony with the laws of nature, with
the teachings of physiology, with the rules of
hygiene, proscribes severely every species of fraud
in the accomplishment of the generative functions. Indeed, this precept is not listened
to. The vascillating reason of man seeks to

substitute itself for the views of Providence; setting itself in defiance of the immutable wisdom of God, does it not imagine that it must re-construct the grand laws which rule the universe? Ridiculous presumption, which gives birth only to error, which sows only the seeds of ruin and death! The man who would, by his ingenuity, derange the admirable combinations of the Creator, who would disturb the law which presides over the conservation and propagation of the species, does not do it with impunity; he must bear the penalty.

Observation confirms this: — In the first place, the culpable end is not always attained. Certain married couples know that nature baffles, sometimes, the most adroit calculations of their ingenuity, that she regains the rights of which they wished to frustrate her. It is remarked that the children, the unexpected products of · these unforseen procreations, feel profoundly the strange perturbations of their conception. They are, in general, feeble, weak, scrofulous, and even monstrous. Furthermore, physicians know that the venereal act, exercised otherwise than under the inspiration of instinct, is a frequent cause of disease for both sexes. In man. the conjugal duty accomplished physiologically, completely, leaves after it a state of comfort, which always results from the satisfaction of an imperious desire. But when the function has been disturbed by culpable pre-occupations, the nervous system is **exalted, and is accompanied by depression, prostra-**

tion, fatigue, and, above all, by a shade of sadness
analogous to a remorse of conscience. By the
repetition of these unnatural acts, derangements in
the health supervene, diseases similar to those produced by solitary onanism, or masturbation—different diseases of the nerves, despondency of the
mind, emaciation, impotence and involuntary
losses — dimness of vision, vertigo or dizziness,
enfeeblement of vital energy, pruritus or excessive
itching, pallor and emaciation, neuralgias of the
head and of the stomach are some of the symptoms
brought on by these practices.

By provoking unsatisfied desires and incomplete
sensations the artifices introduced into the conjugal
act often lead to a profound perturbation in
the genital apparatus of woman. The womb
enters into a state of excitation and congestion,
which is not appeased by the natural crisis, by the
contact and lubrification of the seminal fluid; the
super-excitation persists and is perverted. There
comes to pass then just what will take place if.
after having presented food to a starving man, it is
suddenly withdrawn from his mouth, after having
excited his appetite. These over-excitations not
being calmed, determine, little by little, grave disorders in the uterus; the starting point of varied,
multiple diseases of the nerves, of cramps, strange
hysterical affections, which torment in a cruel manner, and without relaxation, so many married women. Among one hundred women, I have been

able to attribute to Onanism the nervous debility which was the cause of their suffering.

In certain women, conjugal Onanism, by uselessly exciting the procreative faculty, without satisfying the function—without completing it physiologically (as it was intended)—provokes congestions, inflammatory engorgements of the uterus, metritis, leucorrhœa (whites); then granulations, ulcerations of the organ; and finally, according as there is a predisposition, organic affections—grave diseases which are much more common in cities than in the country, where the morals are better preserved. The affections of the organ of gestation have become so frequent in our day, that a writer, unacquainted with medical matters, has felt justified in calling this age the age of womb diseases.

Women cannot have Spermatorrhœa, according to our present classification of diseases: yet, when we study Spermatorrhœa as but symptoms of a lesion or disease of the reproductive function, we can readily see how women may suffer similar lesions without this symptom. I am satisfied, from a considerable experience, that there may be as many cases in women as in men, and that the suffering and danger to mind may be full as great in one as in the other.

The reproductive functions in man and in woman are alike, though the organs differ. There is the same sexual feeling, the same relationship with the emotions and the mind, the same connection with

the spinal cord, and the same relations with all
the vegetative functions through the sympathetic
nervous system. If we study the causes of the
lesion we find that women are quite as much exposed to them as men. We have already seen that
they suffer from self-abuse, not so frequently, it is
true, but quite as severely. And in the marital
relation, they suffer more frequently from excitation of the sexual organs without gratification.
Let this be repeated for years, and the wonder is,
not that we meet with such cases, but that they
are not of more frequent occurrence. Many of
the ills of woman, cloaked under the name of
nervousness, or hysteria, are due to this lesion
of the reproductive function. Thousands of women have endured ill-health, and living a few years
of a sickly, wasted life, have died, without the nature of the lesion and its cause having been suspected. It is not always child-bearing and the
common household cares that bring premature age
and death. These are rarely the cause, as may be
seen in the improved health of women when pregnant. Pregnancy, child-birth and nursing, are
physiological functions, and nature responds to the
call with alacrity. Perpetual gratification of the
lust of a man is unphysiological, and is the cause
of a multitude of maladies attributed to natural
function. It is well to think and talk in plain
English on this subject, for the lesions are so serious and destructive, and the cause so gross, that

they should be brought fairly to view. It may be impossible to rectify the wrong in many cases, but it is possible in a large number, and we illy do our duty as physicians if we do not use our influence in a right direction. Though the lesions are principally nervous, it will do no harm to call attention to the fact that every form of local disease of the uterine organs may be grown from this cause. And, to the more important fact that this abuse must be stopped if we are to have successful results from treatment. Indeed, I have seen severe cases of ulceration of the cervix, that had resisted topical treatment just by incontinence and uncleanliness alone. The disease of the reproductive function may be divided into two classes—one of hyperæmia and increased sensibility of the nervous system and the sexual organs, the other of anæmia, and impaired sensibility. It is well to make this classification of cases, even though the majority may show neither the one nor the other condition as a marked feature. In the one class of cases, the general expression of the body is of contraction—pinched. The features are sharp, the muscles of the face distinctly outlined, the orbicularis orum and palpebrarum (muscles of the mouth and eyebrows) contracted, mouth retracted, eyelids do not close, wings of the nose drawn in, eyes dry, pupils immobile, hair harsh and dry, tongue contracted and incurved, etc. The appetite is variable, digestion poor, bowels inclined to constipation, or constipation alternated with irritative diarrhœa, nutrition impaired, skin parchment-like and dark, etc. You do not have to ask the patient if she suffers—the entire expression is one of suffering. You get a history of pain in back, intense pain in head, pain in every part of the body upon slight exertion, of broken rest, unpleasant sensation of dizziness, oppression about the heart, and uneasiness in the pelvic region. But above all, there is the impairment of conscious life alternating between undue excitation and the apathy of despair, which causes the most intense suffering, though it bears but little relationship to pain. In the opposite cases, the body is expressionless, the movements languid, and the face apathetic. The eyelids are full, dark lines around them, eyes dull, pupils dilated. The tongue is full, pale and slimy, the breath a peculiar sweetish fetor, bowels constipated, digestion and blood-making impaired. She suffers from a sense of fullness and weight in the pelvis, dragging sensations, difficult urination and defacation, is easily exhausted, especially when obliged to be on the feet. This patient sometimes suffers intense pain, but it is the pain of exhaustion, as if nature, wearied with the struggle for life, was about to succomb. In this class, we find atony of the sexual organs. The vulva has lost the fatty tissue, and is soft and relaxed, the vagina dilated, the uterus low, the cervix full, the os dilated and patulous, and from all the mucous surfaces there is an increased secretion. We have a larger number of cases in which the symptoms are the same as described in the lesion of the male. There is marked impairment of the general health, but overshadowing this is the *nervousness*, the desire for seclusion and rest, the downcast look, unsteady eye, languid movement, with the fear of impending danger intensified by sensations of dizziness and oppression about the heart.

FREQUENCY OF SEXUAL INTERCOURSE.

On this question there is as much diversity of opinion as on any other that can be named. The only data on which a philosophical answer can be predicated, is normal instincts; and these, unfortunately, we do not know where to look for. It is easy to lay down a rule by which all may approximate as nearly as possible to physiological propriety—a life in obedience to the laws of life. The more nearly the parties live in accordance with physiological laws, the more nearly normal will be their sexual inclinations, and the less need have they of subjecting their desires to the restraints or control of reason. For those who live riotously; who are constantly goading their sexual passions into abnormal tensity by means of gross food, stimulating viands, and obscene associations, no better rule can be given than, the less indulgence the better.

The majority of young persons unite in matrimony with no education whatever on this subject; and habits, right or wrong, are soon formed, which are apt to be continued through life. I have had patients who had for years indulged in sexual intercourse as often as once in twenty-four hours, and some who have indulged still oftener; of course, the result was premature decay. It was not because these persons were inordinately sensual, or unusually developed in the cerebellum, that they damaged themselves in this way. It was simply because they knew no better. Many a man who would have been a good husband if he had only known how, and who would not for his life, much less for the momentary pleasure it afforded, have endangered the health, or hazarded the happiness of a well-beloved wife, has destroyed her health, happiness, and life (some men several wives successively), by excessive sexual indulgence.

Married men are not always as sensual in character, nor as cruel in disposition, as they seem. With many, sexual intercourse becomes a habit, like eating, working and sleeping; and they indulge in it with nearly the same regularity that they do in their other habits—reckless and thoughtless of its consequences to themselves or their wives. And it is no uncommon thing for the physician to attend an invalid woman for years, whose ailments are chiefly attributable to this habit on the part of her husband. Almost every physician of large practice has a circle of "everlasting patients," whom he visits and prescribes for once a week, on the average, for years: who never get much better at home, but always improve at once when removed to a proper distance from their bosom companions. I do not charge their physicians with remissness in duty in not instructing both parties how to avoid the necessity of employing him professionally, for, generally, physicians are as heedless and as ignorant as the people on this subject. The frequency with which sexual intercourse can be indulged in without serious damage to one or both parties, depends, of course, on a variety of circumstances—constitutional stamina, temperament, habits of exercise, occupation, &c. I am of the opinion that few can exceed the limit of once a week, without serious detriment to health and a premature old age; while many cannot safely indulge oftener than once a month. But as temperance is always the safer rule of conduct, if there must be any deviation from the strictest law of physiology, let the error be on that side. It is a common notion among the public, and even among professional men, that the word *excess* chiefly applies to illicit sexual connection. Of course, whether extravagant in degree or not, all such connection is, from one point of view, *an excess.* But any warning against sexual dangers would be very incomplete if it did not extend to the excesses too often committed by married persons, in ignorance of their ill effects. Too frequent emissions of the life-giving fluid, and too frequent sexual excitement of the nervous system are, as we have seen, in themselves, most destructive. The result is the same, within the marriage bond or without it. The married man who thinks that, because he is a married man, he can commit no excess, however often the act of sexual congress is repeated, will suffer as certainly, and as seriously, as the unmarried debauchee, who acts on the same principle, in his indulgences; perhaps more, certainly from his very ignorance, and from his not taking those precautions, and following those rules which a career of vice is apt to teach the sensualist. Many a man has, until his marriage, lived a most continent life; so has his wife. As soon as they are wedded, intercourse is indulged in night after night; neither party' having any idea that these repeated sexual acts are excesses which the system of neither can bear, and which to the man, at least, is absolute ruin. The practice is continued until health is impaired, sometimes permanently; and when a patient is at last obliged to seek medical advice, he is thunderstruck at learning that his sufferings arise from excesses unwittingly committed. Married people often appear to think connection may be repeated just as regularly and almost as often as their meals. Till they are told of the danger, the idea never enters their heads that they have been guilty of great and almost criminal excess; nor is this to be wondered at, since the possibility of such a cause of disease is, as I have said before, seldom hinted at by the medical man they consult. Some years ago, a young man called on me, complaining that he was unequal to sexual congress, and was suffering from spermatorrhœa, the result of self-abuse. He went under my treatment and was cured, and I lost sight of him for a couple of years, when he returned, complaining that he was scarcely able to move alone. His mind had become enfeebled, there was great pain in the back, and he wished to go under my treatment again. On cross-examining the patient, I found that under the previous treatment he had recovered his powers, and, having subsequently married, had been in the habit of indulging in connection (ever since I had seen him, two years previously) three times a week, without any idea that he was committing an excess, or that his present weakness could depend upon this cause. The above is far from being an isolated instance of men who, having been reduced by former excesses, still imagine themselves equal to any excitement, and when their powers are recruited, to any expenditure of vital force. Some go so far as to believe that indulgence may increase these powers, just as gymnastic exercises augment the force of the muscles. This is a popular error and requires correction. Such patients should be told that the shock on the system, each time connection is indulged in, is very powerful, and that the expenditure of seminal fluid must be particularly injurious to organs previously debilitated. It is by this, and similar excesses, that premature old age and complaints of the generative organs are brought on. In 1860, a gentleman, twenty-three years of age, who had been married two years, came to me in great alarm, complaining that he was nervous and was losing his strength, so that he was unable to manage his affairs. There was pain in his back, the least exertion caused him to perspire, and he had a most careworn countenance. I learnt that he had married a young wife and unconsciously fell into excess, and attempted connection nightly; latterly, erection had been deficient, emission was attended with difficulty, and he felt himself daily less able to discharge what he thought were his family duties. Having read a book of mine, he came to me for relief, and was extremely surprised to find that I considered he had committed excesses, believing that after marriage, frequent intercourse could not be so termed. I at once placed him under treatment, and in a short time he was able again to resume his duties with temperance and due moderation. In 1861, a stout, florid man, about forty-five years of age, was sent to me by a distinguished country practitioner, in consequence of his sexual powers failing him, and one of his testes being smaller than the other. On questioning him, I found that he had been married some

years and had a family. Connection had been indulged in very freely, when, about four years ago,
a feeling of nervousness insensibly came over him,
and about the same time his sexual powers gradually became impaired. The real object, he avowed,
which he had in coming to me was to obtain some
stimulus to increaee his sexual power, rather than
to gain relief for the nervousness and debility under
which he was laboring. Instead of giving remedies
to excite, I placed him under treatment for the
above symptoms, and explained that the lost power
and debility would be overcome as the former
symptoms were removed. Cautioning him at the
same time that his convalescence would depend
upon moderate indulgence.

The lengths to which some married people carry
excesses is perfectly astonishing. I lately saw a
married medical man who told me that for the last
fourteen years, he believed, he had never allowed a
night to pass without having had connection, and
it was only lately, on reading a book of mine, that
he had attributed his present ailments to marital
excesses. The contrast between such a case as this,
where an individual for fourteen years has resisted
this drain on the system, and that of a man who is,
as many are, prostrated for twenty-four hours by
one nocturnal emission, is most striking. All experience, however, shows that, whatever may be the
condition of the nervous system, as regards sexual
indulgences, excesses, sooner or later, tell upon any

frame, and can never be induged in with impunity.
I believe too frequent sexual relations to be much
more common than is generally supposed, and that
they are hardly yet sufficiently appreciated by the
profession as very fruitful causes of ill-health. In
another instance, a medical man called on me, say-
ing he found himself suffering from spermatorrhœa.
There were general debility, inaptitude to work,
and disinclination for sexual intercourse; in fact,
he thought he was losing his senses, and the sight
of one eye was affected. The only way in which
he lost semen was by slight oozing from the penis.
As a boy, he acknowledged having abused himself,
and had been cured; but he married seven years
previously to his visit to me, being then a hearty,
healthy man, and it was only lately that he had
been complaining. In answer to my further inquiry, he stated that since his marriage, he had had
connection two or three times a week, and often
more than once a night. This one fact, I was
obliged to tell him, s fficiently accounted for all
his troubles. The symptoms he complained of
were similar to those we find in persons suffering
from the effects of self-abuse. It is true, that it
may take years to reduce some strong, healthy men,
just as it may be a long time before some boys are
prejudicially influenced, but the ill effects of excesses are, sooner or later, sure to follow. I feel
confident that many of the forms of indigestion,
general ill-health, melancholy, nervous prostration,

diseases of the heart, &c., so often met with, in
adults, depend upon sexual excesses. The directors
of hydropathic establishments must probably
hold some such opinions, or they would not' have
thought it expedient to separate married patients
when they are undergoing the water treatment.
That this cause of illness is not more widely acknowledged and acted on, arises from the natural
delicacy which medical men must feel in putting
such questions to their patients as are necessary to
elicit the facts.

It may very naturally be asked what is meant by
an excess in sexual indulgence. An excess is what
injures health; the same as in any other indulgence.
Few hard-working, intellectual, married men should
indulge in connection oftener than once in seven,
or perhaps ten days. This, however, is only a
guide for strong, healthy men. Generally, I should
say that an individual may consider he has committed an excess, when coitus is succeeded by
languor, depression of spirits, and malaise. This is
the safest definition! Such results should not happen if the male is in good health, and indulges his
sexual desires moderately. No invariable law can
be laid down in a case where so much depends upon
temperament, age, climate and other circumstances,
as well as the health and strength of both parties.
I maintain that in highly civilized communities the
continuance of a high degree of bodily and mental
vigor is inconsistent with more than a very moder-

ate indulgence in sexual intercourse. The still higher principle also holds good that man was not created only to indulge his sexual appetites, and that he should subordinate them to his other duties. It is not the body alone which suffers from excesses committed in married life. Experience every day convinces me that much of the languor of mind, confusion of ideas and inability to control the thoughts, of which some men complain, arise from this cause. Copulation has not alone for its end the generation of beings; it tends also to bring about unification in the nature of the couple, to facilitate the assimilation of the physical and moral qualities of both. The sperm, in fact, has a fecundating action which exercises itself over the entire organism of the woman. It not only fecundates the ovum of the woman, but it fecundates the woman herself, and exercises its action over the entire formative disposition. It is thus that the wife derives many of the qualities of character that she did not possess before her marriage, that her temperament changes, that new habits of nutrition show themselves. If, then, man neglects this general fecundation of woman, he will fail of a powerful means furnished by nature to produce the most intimate unification of man and wife, to give birth to physical and moral sympathies, that indissoluble alliance by reciprocal attachment, those concordances so happy and so desirable in the tastes and aspirations, in the habits and morals. In place of the antique virtues of the

family, do we not see, too often, alas! only coldness, indifference, disunion? Let us go to the bot-
tom of things, and we will discover, ordinarily, this
wound hidden in Onanism. When the husband
and wife violate the sanctity of the conjugal alliance,
when they profane chastity by their intimate acts,
they are seriously wanting in respect for one another; the husband loses his prestige of honor, the
woman her purity of heart. Hence, pernicious
changes are not slow in showing themselves in their
moral relations. Little by little comes on disaffec-
tion, indifference, contempt; then bitterness, resent-
ment, which, increasing one upon another, bring
about those scandalous ruptures, those dramas of
adultery, so frequent in our age.

Bishop Jeremy Taylor says, in his rules for married persons: " In their permissions and license,
they must be sure to observe the order of nature
and the ends of God. *He is an ill husband that
uses his wife as a man treats a harlot,* having no
other end but pleasure. Concerning which our
best rule is, that although in this, as in eating and
drinking, there is an appetite to be satisfied, which
cannot be done without pleasing that desire, yet,
since that desire and satisfaction was intended by
nature for other ends, they should never separate
from those ends, but always be joined with all, or
one of these ends, *with a desire of children, or to
avoid fornication, or to lighten and ease the cares
and sadnesses of household affairs, or to endear*

each other; but never with a purpose, either in act or desire, to separate the sensuality from these ends which hallow it.

"Married persons must keep such modesty and decency of treating each other that they never force themselves into high and violent lusts with arts and misbecoming devices; always remembering that those mixtures are most innocent which are *most simple* and *most natural, most orderly* and *most safe.* It is the duty of matrimonial chastity to be restrained and temperate in the use of their lawful pleasures; concerning which, although no universal rule can antecedently be given to all persons, any more than to all bodies one proportion of meat and drink, yet married persons are to estimate the degree of their license according to the following proportions:—1. That it be moderate, so as to consist with health. 2. That it be so ordered as not to be too expensive of time, that precious opportunity of working out our salvation. 3. That when duty is demanded it be always paid (so far as in our powers and election) according to the foregoing measures. 4. That it be with a temperate affection, without violent transporting desires, or too sensual applications, concerning which a man is to make judgment by proportion to other actions and the severities of his religion, and the sentences of sober and wise persons, always remembering that marriage is a provision for supply of the natural necessities of the body, not for the artificial and procured appe-

tites of the mind. And it is a sad truth that many
married persons, thinking that the floodgates of
liberty are set wide open, without measures or
restraints (so they sail in the channel), have felt the
final rewards of intemperance and lust by their
unlawful using of lawful permissions. Only let each
of them be temperate, and both of them be modest.
Socrates was wont to say that those women to whom
nature hath not been indulgent in good features and
colors should make it up themselves with excellent
manners, and those who were beautiful and comely
should be careful that so fair a body be not polluted
with unhandsome usages. To which Plutarch adds
that a wife, if she be unhandsome, should consider
how extremely ugly she should be if she wanted
modesty; but if she be handsome, let her think how
gracious that beauty would be if she superadds
chastity."   .

IMPOTENCE AND STERILITY.

Impotence consists in the incapacity for copulation, or in the impossibility of exercising the venereal act. Sterility consists in the aptitude of the
organs for procreation, without the power of reproduction. Thus, a person may be impotent but not
sterile, and vice versa. Some writers apply the
term impotence to the male; but such a distinction
is arbitrary and unscientific. The female may be
impotent from mal-formation, and the male sterile
from excessive venery, Onanism, self-pollution, noc-

turnal emissions, spermatorrhœa and diseases of the testicles. A man who is impotent, is necessarily sterile; but a woman may be impotent and not sterile.

There is no subject which distresses most married persons so severely as want of power and strength in the sexual organs; or. which leads to so much domestic unhappiness, .or so often to infidelity. Therefore, it is important to those about to form matrimonial alliances, to know the causes of impotence and sterility.

IN THE MALE.

The causes of manifest impotence of the male are absence of the penis or testicles.

There must be total loss of the penis, as the slightest penetration into the vagina is sufficient for procreation. There may be congenital want of the penis, or it may be partially lost by accident, as by the bites of animals, burns, wounds, or surgical operations; it may be removed close to the pubes, yet the ejaculatory muscles retain their power, and will propel the semen with sufficient, indeed, the natural force, so that it may affect impregnation.

The absence of one or both of the testicles from the scrotum, is no proof of their non-existence in the abdomen; unless the penis be small, the voice puerile, the beard absent, the form delicate, and the whole physical and moral constitution feminine.

It is well known that the testicles may not descend into the scrotum, though they may be fully developed in the abdomen, and perform their functions perfectly; indeed, according to some writers, much better than in the natural situation, but this is questionable.

The destruction of one testicle by contraction or disease is no impediment to procreation, no more than the loss of one eye is to vision. But when both testicles are completely diseased, their secretion is injured or suppressed, and incurable sterility is the consequence. Frequent seminal emissions, or the sudden secretion of semen during such,— resulting from self-abuse—is generally an effectual bar to reproduction. The secreting power of the testes may be very much increased or diminished. The more fluid parts of the spermatic fluid must be absorbed, and the semen must be retained some hours, to effect procreation. Both parties must also have been for some time continent, and likewise in good health.

Both testicles may be removed by castration, yet procreation may be accomplished, as the vesiculæ seminales, or seminal receptacles, may contain at the time of the operation a sufficient quantity of semen for one or two prolific emissions, after which the person will be sterile, but not impotent. Many medical jurists contend that individuals were impotent who were affected with hypospadias; that is, when the urethra opens through any part of its course from its orifice to the scrotum. But it is now proved, that if the opening is so placed that it can enter the vagina, impregnation may follow.

Diminutiveness, or shortness of the penis is no proof of impotence, as the slightest penetration and emission are sufficient for impregnation. I have known several cases of this description, in which the greater part of the organ had been destroyed by sloughing.

Bad stricture of the urethra phymosis, paraphymosis, vegetations, chordee, chancres (diseases described further on in this work), or excessive length of the frænum, cannot be considered absolute causes of impotence, as they can be remedied by surgical operations. Stricture, which nearly closes the canal of the urethra, enlargement of the verumontanum, or prostate gland may prevent the emission of the semen, and cause temporary or permanent sterility. I have been consulted in several cases of the first and second diseases. In two of prostatic disease, the sperm was emitted drop by drop; and in three, both it and the urine were scattered during emission. Nevertheless, all the individuals had offspring.

Large scrotal hernia cause recession of the penis, and may render coition impracticable; but in some cases relief may be afforded. The same observations apply to a large hydrocele; Sarocele or schirrus of the testicle does not cause absolute impotence, as it may be removed by operation; and one testicle remaining is sufficient for procreation.

CONDITIONS NECESSARY FOR COPULATION ON PART OF THE MALE.

Three conditions are necessary on the part of the male for copulation—*erectio, et intromissio penis, cum seminis emissione.*

Impotence in men depends on defect of some one or more of these conditions: *erection, intromission* and *ejaculation of the spermatic fluid* The causes of impotence are more commonly observed in man than in the other sex; and this is easily accounted for, by the greater part the male has to perform in nuptial congress. This is evident from the phenomena which give the virile member the form and disposition proper for erection, the introduction of the organ, and the ejaculation of the semen, which are affected by a violent and complicated action, which requires a concurrence of many indispensable conditions, as the organs not only contract spasmodically to effect the expulsion of the male fluid, but all the body participates in this convulsion at the moment of emission, as if nature, at this instant, forgot every other function.

The causes of impotence and sterility arise from two sources—from malformation of the genitals, or from want of action in them.

IN MAN.

The causes of want of erection may be divided into physical and moral. The physical causes de-

pend on defects of the body and debility. The
moral causes are such as act powerfully on the imagination and produce an atony of the genitals, and
induce an inactivity in organs properly developed.
The genital organs offer two states in the young and
old, which are the frozen zones of existence; the
intermediate state is the torrid zone of life. The
infant has nothing to give, the old has lost all.
Immaturity of age and senescence are often causes
of want of erection. This doctrine, though generally correct, admits of exceptions, as children have
been precociously developed even before the fourth
year, examples of which have often been cited. Then
the frigid or apathetic constitution or a total insen-
sibility to sexual desire, as a result from indulgence
in the solitary vice, self-abuse, is a cause of want of
erection.

A habitude of chastity is another opponent to
erection, such as characterized the ancient fathers
of the desert, and those who, by fasting and other
forms of church discipline, generally, but not always, extinguish certain desires implanted by nature,
but which are, in their opinion, contrary to the purity
that should distinguish those who have made vows
of chastity. The sexual organs of such persons decay, like all other organs whose functions are not
exerted. Long-continued debauchery, whether with
women or by masturbation, will also cause impotence. The impotence caused by the latter excess,
reduces youth to the nullity of old age, **and is too**

often incurable. The most important cause of impotence, is debility of the genital organs, induced by precocious venereal enjoyments; or by the abuse of the sexual function by solitary indulgence or masturbation. In these cases, there is often want of erection, and should a seminal emission take place, the semen does not possess its prolific power. A youth who masturbates himself, and continues the practice as he grows up to manhood, may evince, even after he has arrived at the marriageable age, no disposition towards the other sex. Only their own solitary pleasure can give them any gratification; as far as women are concerned, they are virtually impotent. This solitary vice has a tendency to separate those practicing it from women. At first, of course, it is on the sex that their thoughts dwell, and they embellish an ideal being with all the charms of imaginary perfection; the habit, however, which enslaves them, little by little, changes and depraves the nature of their ideas, and at last leaves nothing but indifference for the very reality of which the image has been so constantly evoked to aid their criminal indulgence. At a later period, when erection is only temporary, and is too incomplete for them to think of sexual intercourse, they abandon themselves with fury to their fatal habit, notwithstanding the almost complete flaccidity in which the erectile tissues are left. At this period, the handsomest woman only inspires these patients with repugnance and disgust, and they ultimately acquire an instinctive aversion—a real hatred for the sex. They dare not always let their feelings on this subject escape them, from fear of their shameful vice being suspected, or the humiliating condition to which they are reduced being discovered; but they lose no opportunity of, as it were, revenging themselves for the repugnance which they believe they produce in woman, and which, in truth, they do inspire, in consequence of the instinctive reciprocity of such feelings that is inevitable. This perversion of the natural excitement, causing temporary impotence, is among one of the saddest pictures which suffering humanity can show. And it may become irremediable, though I have cured a great many cases of those who had almost despaired of being well again.

Every exciting or depressing passion which operates during the act of reproduction, may be a temporary cause of impotence. All causes of debility, whether moral or physical, impede the function of generation. Priapism and satyriasis impede seminal emission. and may be causes of impotence and sterility.

Monstrous enlargements of the penis and scrotum, constant priapism, induced by local or constitutional irritation in some persons, but most frequently the result of a long course of dissipation and libertinism, cause impotence. Many debilitating diseases, such as typhus fever, anasarca, infiltration of the penis and scrotum, falls and blows on the head or spine, are also causes of impotence.

It is known to every well-developed adult, that the influence of the mind is very great on the generative function, and may wholly prevent the completion of the act. If the imagination wanders from the real object of desiring species, impregnation is often, but not always, impeded, and issue seldom follows. When the one party entertains dislike or disgust to the other, or when either allows the mind to be occupied with the image of another individual, the act of generation may be duly performed, and the offspring will bear a strong resemblance to the person who occupied the imagination of the party.

Excessive venery is a frequent cause of want of erection, and impotence. I have been consulted in many cases of this description. This is a frequent cause of want of offspring in young married persons, as well as in those who indulge in a solitary vice. In these cases, the semen may escape without the aid of the ejaculatory muscles, but is imperfect in quality, and is devoid of prolific power until the health is improved. There is generally inflammation of the seminal vesicles in these cases, and seminal debility or spermatorrhœa. The abuse of tobacco is a cause of impotence. The depressing action of tobacco on the sexual powers is very great. It has long been known that when used immoderately it extinguishes the sexual appetite and annihilates the reproductive faculty. I feel confident that the most common, as well as the worst effect of tobacco is that of weakening, and in extreme cases, of destroying the generative functions. It is a prolific source of spermatorrhœa. During one week, lately, I was consulted by three young men suffering from impotence, in all of whom I could trace this weakness to the relaxing, enervating effect of smoking. Happy would it be for them if the abandonment of the vice would at once restore them to health; but no! the evil remains, though the cause is removed—I do not mean remains permanently, because all such cases may be, ultimately, though sometimes slowly, cured. These three cases are merely a few out of many I have seen and treated. The excessive tobacco smoker, one who commences the habit early in life and carries it to excess, if he marry, he deceives his wife and disposes her to infidelity, and exposes himself to ignominy and scorn. If, however, he should have offspring, they generally either are cut off in infancy, or never reach the period of puberty. His wife is often incapable of having a living child, or she suffers repeated miscarriages, owing to the impotence of her husband. If he have children they are generally stunted in growth or deformed in shape; are incapable of struggling through the diseases incidental to children, and die prematurely. And thus the vices of the parent are visited upon the children, even before they reach the second or third generation. I have constantly observed that the children

of habitual smokers are, with very few exceptions,
imperfectly developed in form and size, very ill or
plain-looking, and delicate in constitution. These
imperfections are most manifest in the female offspring, for the procreative inability being chiefly in
the husband, and less in the wife, unless from disgust at his habits, and the female generally deriving
the chief characteristics of form, feature and constitution from the male parent, the female child is
more or less the victim of his vices and debased
habits. If, therefore, ladies sufficiently value their
own happiness, and the health and happiness of
their families, or desire what all desire "who love
their lords," they ought not to marry smokers; nor
should they trust the promises of reformation which
he may make, as they are very seldom kept. Persons who feel that smoking is injurious to them in
any way whatever, or who are desirous of having
instructions to enable them to relinquish the habit,
should have recourse to the best medical advice to
enable them to recover from existing injurious
effects, and to prevent the accession of others which
may supervene at some future period, even although
the habit has been relinquished.

Temporary impotence may arise from moral
causes. There are no facts which so evidently prove
the influence of the moral over the physical state
of man as the phenomenon of erection. A lascivious idea will arise in the midst of our gravest med-
itations; the virile organ will answer to its appeal,

and will become erected, and fit for the function which nature has confided to it; but another thought arising, will instantaneously extinguish, with the most frigid indifference, all amorous transport.

This statement is well exemplified by the effects of the passions. Chagrin, inquietude, and debilitating passions influence the whole economy; jealousy and profound meditation impede the faculty of procreation.

Thus, at the very moment when enjoyment is about to be commenced, too eager desire, the excess of love, the fear of not being loved, timidity, respect, doubt of capability, the fear of being surprised, the shame of excessive modesty on being in the presence of witnesses, antipathy, the continence imposed by real and true love, aversion from filth, and pre-occupations of the mind, are sufficient to oppose erection, and to abate it most suddenly. A newly married man has become suddenly impotent, on discovering his wife to be without hymen, though the absence of this membrane is no proof of unchastity; and a debauchee has as suddenly become impotent on finding the membrane perfect.

It is thus with a literary man, a philosopher, or all those who have a ruling idea, which excites the brain more than the sexual organs. Nevertheless, such individuals are often excessively amorous. Great nervousness, frigidity, a defect in the moral or physical condition, render the act of procreation infecund, and often impossible.

The fear of being impotent is by far the most frequent and powerful cause of this condition. Many individuals suppose there is no physical power when the moral state destroys their desires, and they are impotent as long as they suppose themselves so.

Such is the power of the moral over the physical state of man. Many impotent persons of this class I have cured by quieting the imagination and strengthening the constitution and sexual organs. Some persons labor under moral or temporary, and not under physical or persistent, impotence and are cured by invigorating the general nervous system, and the genital organs.

IMPOTENCE AND STERILITY IN WOMEN.

It has long been held, I think erroneously, that the generative organs of the human female are more complicated than those of the male, and, therefore, that the causes of impotence are more numerous and less apparent than in the other sex. If we examine the genital organs of both sexes, anatomically, we shall find them equally complicated, and possessing an equal adaptation or arrangement of parts, as well as an identity of structure. Thus we find the structure of the penis very similar to that of the external genital orifice and vagina, the fold of the prepuce, the erectile tissue, the openings of the vesiculæ seminales and uterine tubes, and the testes and ovaries, the spermatic chords and the

uterine tubes. We also find the diseases of one sex
as numerous as those of the other; and those who
doubt the assertion, need only to refer to standard
works on diseases of the genito-urinary organs of
the male, for ample proof of this position. Besides,
it would be inconsistent with the wisdom and conformity displayed in all the works of Providence,
that one sex should have more organs for the per-
petuation of the species than the other.

A cause of impotence in women may be a mal-
formation or disease of the sexual organs. This
may be apparent or obscure; an apparent cause
may be obliteration of the external sexual organs,
both soft and bony, absence of the vagina and
uterus, and great deformity of the pelvis, with numerous diseases of the external and internal genitals. The vagina and uterus have been found to
consist of a dense fleshy substance, and the vagina
has been partially closed by a similar growth. It
may be absent, unusually small, impervious from
adhesions, tumors, or a frænum passing across
above the hymen, or it may be filled with a fleshy
production. If too narrow, it may be dilated with
a bougie, or a sponge tent, and where unattended
to, must be divided by incision, to admit of coition,
or the passage of the infant—the orifice may co-
here after conception. There is sometimes a great
congenital confusion of parts—so much so, that
it would be tedious to describe them. The vaginal
canal may be totally or partially obliterated; and

in such cases an operation is impractible, and impotence absolute. The vagina has opened into the bladder, into the rectum, on to the anterior wall of the abdomen, and pregnancy has occurred.

Inflammation, ulceration, cancer, ossification, calcareous deposit, or tumors in any of these organs, may be the cause of sterility. In fact, any disease of the female genitals, attended with such constitutional disturbance, may be considered a temporary cause of sterility.

Many women never have a pleasurable sensation in sexual commerce; in others, the venereal orgasm is slight and of rare occurrence; in some, it is as it should be, and intensely pleasurable. We find cases in which there is no reciprocity in the sexual act. The man is very excitable, and has the venereal orgasm before the female organs are in a condition to respond, and the woman never has any enjoyment from the act. In such cases, the woman's health will sometimes suffer severely, and the nervous symptoms of spermatorrhœa will be developed. In some cases, there is a natural coldness on the part of the woman; it may be from enfeebled innervation, which can be remedied by treatment.

This want of sexual power may be but the expression of imperfect ovulation, and we then direct our means to an improvement in this respect.

In the majority of cases, the habit of Onanism has been the cause of pleasure in sexual congress and sterility. It appears that nothing but the morbid excitement produced by the baneful practice can give any sexual gratification, and that the natural stimulus fails to cause any pleasure whatever. So ruinous is this practice of solitary vice, both in the one and other sex—so difficult is it to give it up, that I fear it may be carried on even in married life, where no excuse can be devised, and may actually come to be preferred to the natural excitement.

Venereal excesses engender satiety, just as certainly as any other indulgences, and satiety is followed by indifference and disgust.

If the natural excesses of masturbation take place early in life, before the subjects who commit them have arrived at maturity, it is not surprising that we meet with women whose sexual feelings, if they ever existed, become prematurely worn out.

Vaginismus, or spasm of the vagina, may prevent sexual congress. The sexual organs are so excitable, that the thought of the act causes intense congestion, and contraction of the muscles of the perineum, or the slightest touch is sufficient to occasion the spasm of the muscles and intense sensibility of surface. In some cases, this spasm of the structures is most intensely painful, and lasts long after the cause has subsided.

Sterility is not dependent, in most cases, upon inability to perform the sexual act, in either sex. The reproductive function in the female is, to a considerable extent, independent of sexual feeling, and conception will occur when the woman has been wholly passive, and has no sensation of sexual orgasm. To a more limited extent, this is true of man, and he may beget children without the marked pleasurable sensations that the majority experience. In the female, sterility is most frequently dependent upon imperfect ovulation, rather than structural wrong in the reproductive canals, though this is the cause in some cases. This imperfection may, or may not be, marked by menstrual irregularities.

Imperfect ovulation may depend upon undue excitation of the ovarian nerves, and determination of blood, and when there is impaired innervation and congestion.

Dysmenorrhœa is not an uncommon symptom in sterility of women. It may be dependent upon stricture of the os internum or cervical canal, but in most cases it is a functional lesion. There is undue excitement of the sympathetic and spinal nerves distributed to the uterus, and in most cases, this is associated with an exaltation of the semi-erectile tissue of the organ, which prevents the free escape of the menstrual blood.

Congestion of the lower segment of the uterus, may, or may not be, associated with pain, and yet be a cause of sterility. Examination shows the neck or cervix enlarged, with a peculiar tumid, waxy appearance of tissue and enfeebled circulation, whilst the touch gives a sense of fullness, with impaired circulation and nutrition. The mouth of the uterus may be patulous and open, with a free secretion from the cervical canal, or it may be constricted.

Incompatibility of temperament may be a cause of sterility. In every locality, instances may be observed of healthy couples who have no children. Both husband and wife have healthy reproductive organs, and there are neither physical nor functional reasons why they should not be fertile. In many cases, a prior or second marriage has been fruitful in both parties, proving conclusively that the wrong is of neither party as an individual, but an incompatibility of the two. And it seems a fact, that persons approximating to the same temperament generally are sterile.

SEXUAL PATHOLOGY.

PART SECOND.

VENEREAL DISEASES

These are the most widely spread and afflicting diseases of all those with which the human race has been visited. Their ravages are truly frightful, and the unhappy patient is rendered doubly miserable by the dread of exposure. The nature of venereal disease has been a subject of dispute ever since it was first observed; but the most celebrated of European and American authors now agree that in all its forms, it is the consequence of inoculation by a specific virus, which may, however, and is, often taken into the system innocently. I do not believe that contact with a diseased person is necessary. In the male it is often developed through excessive use of the organs, particularly where they have been weakened by past abuse. Constant excitement of the seminal vessels produces irritation and genuine gonorrhœal discharge; if the system be radically healthy, this soon disappears, but when the body is in a depraved condition, the evil increases and all the consequences of genuine gonorrhœa may be developed. The same will ensue in like cases, from a connection with a woman who has the fluor albus (an acrid secretion). There is little doubt that the venereal virus was first engendered in this way.

Females, too, may contract the disease without intercourse with a depraved male organism. Copulation, during the term of menstruation, or while suffering from fluor albus or ovarian disease, will often cause extensive precipitations of pus from an over irritated mucous membrane.

The infection has also often been caught without bodily contact with any one. Young boys and girls have often been known to take the virus from a water closet, or from the use of towels or bedclothes after those suffering from syphilis. We need not enlarge on this topic. We mention these things only for the purpose of warning to those who may be suffering from it, and refuse to seek medical advice, because they do not conceive it possible for them to be suspected as not having been guilty of promiscuous intercourse. Whenever derangement of the sexual organs occurs—no matter how slight—a competent medical man should at once be consulted, as delays may prove the ruin of the tender vessels which compose the sexual organs, and ultimately of the whole frame. Never are delays more dangerous than in such a case.

GONORRHŒA.

Gonorrhœa is a contagious purulent inflammation of the urethra and vagina, with occasional

extension to other mucous surfaces by contamination with the discharge from the urethra.
Certain complications also attend it now and then;
as rheumatoid inflammation of the joints and eyes,
and synovial bursæ. The chief causes of gonorrhœa or urethritis are contagion, and excessive irritation of the urethra through sexual excitement
and other causes. Acrid discharges in the female,
which have not risen from contagion, may excite urethritis in the male. Thus, the condition of the
individual is much concerned in his contracting or
escaping urethritis.

The seat of the disease is at first the urethra as
far as the fossa navicularis, thence it travels down
to the bulbous and membranous parts, leaving
patches of the mucous membrane here and there
inflamed. In certain cases, it extends to the prostate and cellular tissue about the urethra, to the
neck of the bladder and the epididymis.

The anatomical changes in the mucous membrane
are general uniform congestion in the acute stage;
as the inflammation subsides, the surface is marked
by patchy redness, arborescent and punctiform congestion, fine granulations reaching to the size of
warts, induration, and contraction of the mucous
membrane, which cause stricture and irregularity
of the passage.

The symptoms commence generally, as patients
state, within twenty-four hours after suspicious
coitus, beginning then first to notice strange sen-

sations along the urethral canal, such as increased heat, irritation, itching, &c.

There is scarcely any period of incubation or absolute dormancy. The virus commences its action almost from the moment it is deposited. The disease, at first, consists of a little discharge from the lips of the meatus urinarius, which are glazed over, or perhaps become patulous, red, and slightly tumefied.

On squeezing the organ, the morbid exudation slides along the canal, and runs down upon the frænum in thick, transparent, ropy masses.

These symptoms constitute the initial stage of gonorrhœa. By the second or third day from the first appearance of the mucous secretion, the inflammation acquires more intensity. The discharge becomes more abundant, and instead of being merely a glutinous substance, it is changed to purulent matter—is more consistent—of a greenish-yellow tinge, and emits a disagreeable, nauseous odor, wholly different from that of ordinary pus.

The effluvium is sometimes so strong and impressive on the olfactories, that the practitioner recognizes the nature of the case before the patient tells what ails him. This disgusting symptom, when once noticed, will ever afterwards be remembered, and needs no further description. By the time the secretion becomes puriform, the patient begins to complain of ardor urinæ, and has frequent calls to urinate. The inflammation diminishes the

normal calibre of the urethral canal, and consequently the stream of urine is small and flattened.
The shaft of the penis is enlarged, and the glans
assumes a dark red color, is tender to the touch,
and very likely excoriated. If the inflammation be
limited to the fossa navicularis, as it usually is for.
several days, the pain in micturition will also be
confined to this spot. If the organ be pressed between the thumb and finger, the patient will complain of being hurt at this part, and the physician
will here also detect distinct induration and abnormal thickening of the urethra. If the disease
advance, and the bulbous portion of the canal be
implicated in the inflammatory process, pain will
be felt along the perinæum, especially when the
patient undertakes to walk about. If the prostate
become affected, the distress will be felt farther
back; there will be pain, and an uncomfortable
degree of heat and throbbing about the rectum,
with tenesmus and incontinence, or retention of
urine.

Another quite frequent and annoying symptom
is the occurrence of involuntary and painful erections at night, which interfere with, or wholly
prevent, quiet repose.

At this juncture, still other morbid phenomena
will arise, unless those already mentioned are subdued. Pains in the head, in the lumbar and inguinal regions will set in; the tongue will be thickly
coated. the pulse accelerated. the mouth parched

with thirst, and the skin hot and dry. Gonorrhœa presents various degrees of severity in different subjects. The first attack is generally attended with the most acute symptoms, especially if the patient be young and plethoric, or of a scrofulous diathesis. In the latter class, the constitutional disturbance is sometimes of an alarming type. Extensive abscesses form in some portion of the genital organs, or in their immediate neighborhood, accompanied with inflammatory fever and irritation of the nervous system, and the patient's life is endangered. In those who are liable to eczema and other eruptions of the skin, the disease is prone to assume a chronic character from the beginning, and is then difficult of cure. Sometimes, notwithstanding judicious medical attention, the complaint progresses steadily, from day to day, for several weeks, the discharge increasing in quantity, with corresponding augmentation of the other symptoms. In such cases, if the previous habits of the patient can be ascertained, it will generally be found that he has led an irregular life, or that he is susceptible to inflammatory affections of the mucous membrane; and the system refuses to respond to the usual remedies.

Persons who have had several fresh attacks of this malady suffer for a longer time from each successive one, although the symptoms do not acquire so high a degree of intensity as they do in the first gonorrhœa.

Gonorrhœa often subsides into a chronic form, and terminates in gleet or stricture. The amount of discharge is reduced to two or three drops in the twenty-four hours. In some cases, it is noticed only in the morning; in others, the orifice of the urethra is constantly moistened with it or its lips are sealed together a greater portion of the time, in consequence of the drying up of the exudation. The fluid is of a serous or mucous character. If pus globules be present, they separate into a pellicle by themselves, and leave a small, yellow stain upon the patient's linen.

Sometimes the gleet is intermittent. It will disappear for several days, and then, in consequence of some imprudence, will again return. Any irregularity or indulgence on the part of the patient, or any impropriety in treatment, may result in a long establishment of this troublesome disease.

GLEET.

This is a frequent sequel of an obstinate gonorrhœa unsuccessfully treated or wholly neglected. The discharge is, as I have said, slight. Sometimes only a drop or two is noticed about the meatus urethræ, in the morning.

The orifice is smeared with a ropy, tenacious serous or mucous fluid, partially dried, perhaps, upon the lips, and slightly impeding the free exit of the stream of urine, when it first arrives at this part. Some patients have an oozing of matter, amounting to five or six drops in the twenty-four hours. Sometimes several days will intervene and no discharge be noticed; but if the patient indulge in any imprudence in diet, severe exercise, sexual intercourse, or anything which tends to excite the organs, the gleet will very probably reappear.

The most common seat of this disease is in the vicinity of the membranous or prostatic portion of the urethra; the lesion, however, is sometimes situated in, or near, the fossa navicularis, as in acute urethritis. It is generally easy to determine when it is seated at the latter point: for if it be, moderate squeezing of the glans penis will force the matter out at the orifice of the urethra, whereas this cannot be so readily done if the discharge proceeds from a portion of the canal farther back. Sometimes the locality may be ascertained by pressing the integument along the urethra. The patient will complain of being hurt when the diseased spot is reached. Occasionally, a preternatural redness and turgescence of the lips of the urethra remain after the discharge has ceased. This deviation from the healthy appearance is, of itself, an affair of but little moment. It is, however, indicative of a more profound abnormal condition, which may still be lurking in the mucous lining of the canal, in Cowper's glands, or in the prostate, either or all of which parts may have been, at some period of the disease, concerned in the production of the morbid secretion, and may still be the seat

of a sub-acute inflammation; and so long as this
continues, the patient is liable to a relapse from
the most trivial excess or imprudence. I have
examined with the microscope numerous specimens
of true gleety matter. In instances it consists of
large, delicate, well defined epithelial cells and free
nuclei, which remain entire after the other portions
of the morbid product are decomposed and broken
up into mere shreds and amorphous granules. In
most instances, I have found pus-globules, although
seldom in abundance. If the individual indulge in
any excess, and thus augment the local inflammatory action, a corresponding increase of pus-globules
can be detected. So a gleet may be aggravated by
any cause which produces urethral irritation, and
can be readily transformed into a gonorrhœa. A
hearty meal, alcoholic stimulants, free sexual indulgence, violent exercise, or a long ride, may bring on
a copious, purulent discharge, attended by swelling,
scalding in passing the urine, and all the other
symptoms of acute gonorrhœa. Some writers on
venereal regard the discharge peculiar to gleet as
not infectious, but, in my opinion, this is a grave
error, and calculated to work great mischief. It is
indeed true that men suffering from gleet have been
known to have connection with their wives for years,
with impunity, but where contagion ceases and im-
munity begins no one can tell. And if the discharge is at some times innocuous, a few hours'
sexual indulgence may effect a complete change in

this respect. Long continued gleet is about certain, sooner or later, to cause sexual debility, inability, or nervous debility, with all its train of evils, and therefore requires diligent care on the part of the patient, and good skill on the part of the physician.

This disease may be caused, also, by disorder and disease of the bladder or kidneys, and by various affections of the prostate gland. It is often maintained by a state of general debility, or by scrofulous, rheumatic, or gouty diathesis. This general debility is a fruitful source of the persistency of gleet, and the disease is frequently very intractable in persons of broken down constitutions.

STRICTURE.

When a gonorrhœa or gleet resists treatment for a length of time, there is ample reason for suspecting the presence of stricture, which keeps up the discharge. One of the earliest symptoms of permanent stricture is a slight discharge from the urethra. This discharge is not a constant symptom, but is present in a majority of cases.

Generally, the patient cannot retain his water as long as usual, and sometimes is obliged to make quite an effort before the urine appears, and the stream may be variously distorted; sometimes it is flattened; at other times spiral, forked or divided into two streams, or the last drops may fall at his feet, with generally more or less pain. This is caused by chronic inflammation, leading to plastic deposits in the mucous membrane at some part of the urethra, or in the sub-mucous tissue, or else ultimately extending to them and the corpus spongiosum. In the initiatory stages, it is probable that there it some muscular contraction resulting from the frequent passing of the urine over an inflamed and slightly thickened mucous membrane, and this occurring at the time that the plastic deposit is becoming organized, results in the formation of a more or less wide circular band around the urethra, narrowing its canal. The persistence of the cause, and the additional cause resulting from the narrowing of the passage, the extension of the inflammation and deposit into the sub-mucous tissues, and possibly the effects of careless instrumental interference, ultimately result in so close a contraction of this band, and such an indurated condition of it and adjacent tissues, that urine can no longer be expelled, excepting after long waiting, much effort, or in very bad cases only in a few drops at a time.

BALANITIS.

Balanitis signifies inflammation of the surface of the glans penis, the mucous membrane of the prepuce, the glandulæ odoriferæ, and the follicles that surround the corona. The disease is known sometimes, as external gonorrhœa, spurious or false gonorrhœa. The inflammation is attended with more or less muco-purulent discharge, with or without superficial excoriations. If the disease be con-

fined to the *prepuce*, it is called *posthitis.* But, as
in most cases, all the tissues just named are involved, the term balanitis is sufficiently suggestive
of the complaint. The liability of men to this disorder depends in some degree upon the amount of
preputial integument, with which the parts are naturally endowed; and in this particular, very great
differences are found. In some men, the prepuce
is very long, but in others it is of remarkable brevi-
ty—hardly sufficient to conceal any portion of the
glans, which, with them, always remains in nearly
the same condition as if circumcision had been performed.

The glandulæ odoriferæ, with their short excretory ducts, situated behind the glans, are disseminated
much more plentifully in some men than in others;
varying numerically, from ten to one hundred; and
while they are designed by nature to perform an
important emunctory function, analagous to that
of the sweat glands of the skin, they are at the
same time subservient to the protection and healthy
condition of the parts in the immediate neighborhood, upon the surface of which they constantly
pour out an oily, lubricating fluid. But, if this oily
material be allowed to accumulate, and to become
partially concrete, it may, and frequently does,
prove a source of irritation and inflammation. This
accumulation is much more rapid and difficult of
prevention if the glans be invested by a preter-nat-
urally elongated prepuce, than is the case where the

glans are naked, or covered by a foreskin of normal length and easy of retraction.

The existence of the prepuce is the principal predisposing cause of balanitis.

The exciting causes of the complaint are numerous. Impure sexual congress is at the head of the list. The menstrual fluid, leucorrhœa, masturbation, and inattention to cleanliness will oftentimes produce it.

If it be the result of intercourse with an infected female, the symptoms generally begin to show themselves in a day or two after exposure. The period of incubation is shorter than in cases of urethral inflammation. The first warning of the trouble is a slight tingling or smarting sensation in the prepuce or glans; the prepuce becomes very tender and swollen; and if it be drawn back upon the glans, the latter will exhibit inflammatory action, more or less intense; and at a later period, if nothing be done to check the morbid process, a discharge of puriform fluid will take place from the glans, near the frænum. There is scalding in urinating. If the trouble arise from uncleanliness, it is more gradual in its development; the symptoms declaring themselves more and more manifestly as the acrid sebaceous product is allowed to accumulate. The muco-purulent matter, mingled with the natural secretion from the parts, is sometimes very abundant, and if the preputial orifice be narrow, and the escape of the fluid obstructed, will sometimes give rise to a sort of abscess; and it may be necessary to puncture the prepuce for the purpose of evacuating it. If phymosis complicate the balantis, and the case be neglected, or injudiciously conducted, sloughing of the prepuce may take place, and the glans be seized with severe inflammation; and this morbid action may extend to the lymphatics of the penis and of the inguinal region.

PHYMOSIS.

Phymosis is the condition a long, tight prepuce assumes when inflammation attacks the glans beneath it. The foreskin swells with œdema, and often sloughs away, from the circulation being arrested by the swelling.

PARAPHYMOSIS.

When there is great constriction and narrowing of the prepuce from inflammation, it frequently happens that if this covering be pulled back behind the glans, it cannot again be brought forward to its normal position over this portion of the organ. It remains retracted, forming a band or ligature around the part just behind the corona, and occasioning strangulation analagous to that which takes place in intestinal hernia. This condition of the penis is known as *paraphymosis.*

Infiltration into the integument takes place rapidly on either side of the stricture; and the glans likewise is distended with blood, and painful. There seems to be no power in the system to con-

trol the local inflammatory process that has been
awakened; and which, if not checked by judicious
management, will very likely result in a partial or
total destruction of some of the tissues.

ORCHITIS.

The testicles are connected by continuity of tissue
with the mucous lining of the urethra, through the
medium of the vasa deferentia; and when inflammation has reached that part of the urethra in
which these minute, intermediate canals terminate,
it readily enough finds its way into them, and
rapidly pursues its march until it arrives at the
convolutions of the epididymis, where its further
progress is usually arrested. This appendix of the
testis receives and retains the principal force of
the morbid action, and thus serves as a wall of
protection to the parenchyma of the gland itself.

Sometimes the enemy overleaps this barrier and
attacks the testis proper. In all cases, there is a
general and sudden swelling—a swelling of the testicle, as we term it—but this enlargement is produced by the presence of lymph and serum within
the tunica vaginalis.

The epididymis is, after all, the chief seat of the
disease in most instances. The old theory of me-
tastasis, or the sudden translation of the inflammation from the urethra to the testicle, is not enti-
tled to much favor. It is extremely questionable
whether anything of the kind ever takes place in

gonorrhœal orchitis. The inflammation, in a majority of subjects, may be traced advancing along the vas deferens to the epididymis; or the morbid action may seize upon the latter without involving the vas deferens. In nearly all cases of orchitis, the pain and urethral discharge diminish very considerably, especially during the early stage of the testicular affection.

The attack commences with a sense of increased weight in the testis, with a dull pain along the course of the spermatic chord, in the perineum, in the groin, and in the lumbar region. In a few hours, the epididymis becomes swollen at the lower portion, or tail, as it is called—is hard, knotty and tender to the touch; the patient can scarcely tolerate any covering upon that side of the scrotum, or bear to have it come in contact with the thigh. He feels most comfortable when he holds it in his hand. In two or three days, if not arrested, the inflammation reaches the tunica vaginalis; and the general tumefaction which preserves the natural, oval contour of the testicle, increases to the size of a hen's egg. The pain, which in the beginning was of a dull, aching description, soon becomes more absolute, especially when the patient attempts to assume the erect posture. There is great irritation in the bladder, and a constant desire to urinate. The distress about the loins, hips, and scrotum is sometimes excruciating. As the disease advances to its culmination, the surface of the scrotum, which invests the gland, participates in the inflammation—becomes red, hot, thickened, and œdematous. Generally, the constitutional disturbance is not severe; occasionally, it assumes a very serious character. Sometimes the patient suffers from extreme nausea, and perhaps vomits freely; the tongue is coated; there is great thirst; quick pulse; and all the symptoms maintain their activity for eight or ten days, by which time they usually become milder. The gonorrhœa diminishes or wholly subsides for the time being; and when the order of events is reversed in regard to the orchitis—that is, when the symptoms begin to be less severe, and convalescence from the scrotal trouble is fairly commenced—the gonorrhœa generally reappears. Now and then the urethral discharge is not affected in any way by the swollen condition of the testicle, and even where the swelling has gone on increasing to the size of the fist; and what is still more singular, instances have been known where the testicles have swollen and yet the discharge has become more profuse than before.

In some feeble constitutions, the symptoms are moderate in degree, slow of development, and long in duration.

Such cases are less easy of management than those in which an intensity of symptoms prevails. A trivial circumstance, such as carelessness on the part of the patient, or deviation from the proscribed line of treatment, will be sufficient to interrupt his

progress towards a cure, and, perhaps, will provoke
an unfortunate relapse. In some such way, the
malady may be transformed into a chronic orchitis
or epididymitis, which may harass the patient more
or less for many months, or even years.

HERPES PRÆPUTIALIS.

This vesicular affection is of frequent occurrence.
Men who have a long, superabundant preputial
membrane are more liable to be troubled with the
eruption than others. Those who are familiar with
its appearance in the different stages of its existence.
and who have much practical experience in its treatment, may consider that it is so insignificant, and
so unlike any syphilitic sore, that it is hardly enti-
tled to consideration in this place.

But a correct diagnosis of the eruption is a matter of no little consequence; for an error or confusion here will lead to improper treatment, to say
nothing of the moral bearings immediately connected with the subject.

Patients who have contracted herpes upon the
penis in consequence of sexual intercourse, or who
have suffered from it as a concomitant or sequel of
gonorrhœa, have occasion to apply to the physician
for the purpose of obtaining his opinion in the
premises. And in some instances, herpetic eruptions located upon the foreskin have been treated as
chancrous products. Such cases have presented
themselves to my notice, and although not frequent,

they justify the appropriation of a few pages to the
exanthem in question.

The most common seat of the eruption is along
the border of the prepuce, where the external and
internal surface meet. At first, a sensation of heat
and smarting, accompanied with considerable itching, draws the attention of the patient to the part
upon which the eruption is about to be evolved.
Upon inspection, he notices that it is slightly thickened and suffused with a preternatural redness;
and if he merely touch it with his fingers, he in-
duces a higher degree of itching, and rubs it with
the expectation of appeasing the sensation. In a
few hours he perceives, if he looks, an aggregation
of some dozen or twenty points closely crowded
together, and, on careful examination, discovers
that these pimples are filled with a transparent, watery fluid. They are the vehicles of herpes præputialis. They are about the size of a common pin's
head, and have been compared to so many transparent glass beads reposing on a red base. Instead
of one group or cluster, two or three may appear
simultaneously. They are not inclined to enlarge
the area they occupy. But have nearly the same
dimensions in the latter stages which they had at
first. Instead of appearing on the confines of the
preputial orifice, as mentioned above, the eruption
may arise at a little distance from it, either on the
mucous or cuticular surface of this membrane. In
two or three days, the contents of these globular

vesicles lose their transparency, and are slightly
turbid; and in four or five days, the matter becomes
· puriform.   The walls of the individual vesicles
break away, and the eruption is then confluent. Next,
dessication ensues, forming a thin, delicate, incrustation, which in two or three days is cast off, and
brings to view a smooth, raw, florid spot, amounting to little more than an abrasion; or, if it be an
ulcerated surface, it is of the most superficial kind,
and has no hardened base as in syphilitic ulcers.
When the complaint is situated on the inner surface
of the prepuce, the inflammation is generally quite
severe.   The vesicles are usually a little larger than
when developed on the external surface.

The serous exudation of herpes passes rapidly into
a lactescent state; the membrane or sac containing
it is easily ruptured, and excoriations are produced,
which may be mistaken for venereal ulcerations.
But the speedy development and progress of the
eruption, the level of the exposed surface after the
incrustations have fallen off, with the adjacent
healthy tissue, and the ordinarily transient duration
of the affection, are entirely in contrast with the
true venereal sore.   I must here remark, that, if
the herpetic action take place on the inner surface
of the prepuce, no incrustation or scab is formed,
in consequence of the constant moisture of the
parts, and their protection from the air.   If the
eruption be not seen by the physician until five or
six days after its first appearance—by which time

incrustations may have formed on the skin, or the secretion have passed into a sero-purulent state—and if its antecedents indicate that the patient has been exposed, then it will not be an easy matter to say whether the affection be follicular chancres, or simply herpetic.

The eruption of herpes, when situated upon the foreskin, is quite evanescent, if not injudiciously tampered with. It runs its course in eight or ten days, and then, in most cases, all is over.

Occasionally it becomes chronic, and extremely difficult to cure.

Sometimes numerous minute vesicles are seen clustered on the mucous surface of the prepuce, along the fossa just behind the corona glandis, and forming a cincture around the organ. The accompanying inflammation is moderate; and when the vesicles burst, there is seldom any disposition to assume an ulcerative process, and there is a total want of depth to the sore.

The foregoing description gives, in the main, the characteristic features presented by herpes præputialis, whether situated on the external or internal surface. The complaint derives its chief importance from two facts: one is, that it is too apt to be regarded by the patient, and sometimes by the medical adviser, as syphilitic; and the other, that a man having it, or being predisposed to it, is more liable, *cæteris paribus*, to contract a venereal affection than one who has no such herpetic tendency.

IRRITABILITY OF THE BLADDER.

In some cases of gonorrhœa which become chronic, a certain amount of irritability of the bladder is induced, which often requires medical treatment. Persons of a nervous temperament are particularly liable to suffer from this affection, while those of a robust, sanguineous constitution are more disposed to cystitis or inflammation of the bladder. In irritability of this viscus, the mucous membrane becomes morbidly sensitive; and the presence of the urine is quite insupportable. The patient complains of a sense of uneasiness in the lumbar region, about the verge of the anus, at the extremity of the penis, and above the pubes; he is continually haunted with a desire to pass urine, and unable to endure the smallest accumulation of this fluid. It is seldom that he suffers much pain anywhere, but his nervous system is wrought up to a state of constant excitement. He loses all relish for food, and sleep departs from him; and if these abnormal conditions are not removed, the general complexion of the symptoms will simulate those of cystitis, or what is still worse, the latter disorder will actually set in. In mere irritability of the bladder, the system is rarely affected; whereas, in inflammation, it is always involved. This is the rule, and should be borne in mind in forming the diagnosis. Simple irritation may also be known by the absence of that profuse secretion of mucous, which is a prominent characteristic of catarrhus vesicæ. In the latter affection, immense quantities of thick, semi-transparent, tenacious mucous, and coagulable lymph, accumulate in the bladder, and frequently block up the urethral canal, so as to impede, or wholly prevent, the flow of urine. Sometimes the complaint extends to the ureters and kidneys, which contribute a share of the secretion that is produced in such extraordinary quantities.

In irritation, the urine is free from any admixture of blood; in inflammation, it is more or less deeply tinged. In inflammation, there is constant and severe distress in the rectum, with a sensation of heat and throbbing in the part as well as along the course of the perineum; and if the surgeon make gentle pressure upon the supra-pubic region, the patient will complain of lancinating pain, which is not the case when the viscus is merely in an irritable state. In inflammation of the vesical mucous membrane, the symptoms, both local and constitutional, are all of a much more grave and intense character than those which prevail in uncomplicated irritation.

An acute attack of irritation occasionally passes into a chronic state, and may lead to suspicion that a calculus exists in the bladder; and this idea may suggest to the surgeon the importance of introducing the sound; whereas, if this instrument be used, the chances are that it will excite inflammation in the organ, which has thus been needlessly explored. The patient's condition goes on from bad to worse.

No stone is found; and a little reflection upon what has passed, and a more abiding and deliberate attention to what is present, will now enable the surgeon to form a correct diagnosis of the case. To such a course of procedure, with such results as are here mentioned, the annals of surgery abundantly testify.

The most salient points of difference between irritability of the bladder and a calculus within its cavity, may be summed up in a few words.

In the latter disease, the moment of the patient's greatest suffering is after the last jet of urine has escaped from the meatus urinarius; whereas, if he have only an irritable bladder, the time of his greatest distress is before the urine is evacuated; and the amount of pain experienced will be in proportion to the quantity of urine contained in the bladder. If the physician has a knowledge of these simple facts, he will have no occasion to introduce an instrument for the purpose of resolving doubts and arriving at a true diagnosis.

When irritability of the bladder assumes a chronic character, it is one of the most formidable and dreadful maladies that can befall the patient. He is compelled to keep aloof from society, and his life of seclusion is also a life of almost unremitting torment. If irritation and inflammation coexist, as they sometimes do, the latter, being the more important of the two, should occupy our chief attention.

EXCORIATIONS.

Simple abrasion of some portion of the glans penis, or of the mucous or cutaneous surface of the prepuce, is not an infrequent accident resulting from sexual congress. The injury takes place where there is a want of co-aptation in the relative size of the organs, or where the parties engage in their amative embraces in an impetuous manner. The most frequent locality of the disease is near the frænum, or just behind the corona, among the glandulæ odoriferæ. Although it is one of the non-specific affections incidental to the venereal act, it is very apt to be viewed by the patient with alarm, as being syphilitic. The excoriation is sometimes on the free edge of the prepuce, especially when the latter is long and narrow, and does not readily retract behind the glans. Such a prepuce is liable to receive the brunt of the effort; and the seat of injury is along the line of union between the two surfaces—oftener than elsewhere; and least in frequency the lesion is met with upon the dorsum of the glans and on the external surface of the prepuce, a few lines from the orifice.

When situated within the preputial cavity, the abrasions, if neglected, sometimes assume an appearance closely allied to chancres. They ulcerate, occasion little or no pain or smarting, and are attended with only a moderate inflammation. If early treated, they can be easily cured; but if allowed to take their own course for a week or two, uninfluenced by remedial means, the sores or ulcerations which form upon the abraded spots are extremely reluctant to heal,—not on account of any peculiar, bad quality, inherent in them, but partly because of the structures in which they are situated, and partly from the fact that the secretions to which the diseased surface is exposed, keep up a morbid irritation.   Generally, there is but one irritated patch.

Ulcerations, resulting from abrasions of the cutaneous surface of the prepuce, bear less resemblance to chancres than those situated within the orifice. They are on a plane with the adjacent healthy integument, and of course do not present the elevated, sharp, perpendicular edges which characterize chancres; nor have they any indurated base, which many chancres have.   They are irregular in form and size.   After the excoriation has healed, the integument remains quite tender for some time; and a slight cause, such as friction of the part against the clothing, is sufficient to awaken the injury anew. Such relapses are not uncommon, and they are generally worse than the original attack.   The surface of the excoriation is larger, and the morbid action now reestablished is more difficult to subdue. It sometimes assumes a chronic type, and gives rise to a sympathetic bubo in the groin.

VEGETATIONS.

These morbid excrescences were once, but are not now, regarded as the product of the syphilitic poison. They are sometimes the result of irritation from the deposit of gonorrhœal matter; and sometimes they are generated by the combined agency of moisture, heat, and filth, especially in uncleanly females, who may or may not have some vaginal discharge at the same time. They differ in appearance, and sundry terms have been employed to designate them, which are not necessary to repeat. The situations in which they are chiefly found, are the meatus urinarius, the glans, the mucous membrane of a narrow prepuce, and at the junction of the two preputial surfaces; when they select the latter site and are allowed to remain, they fill up the orifice so as to impede the escape of urine, and otherwise interfere with the functions of the penis. In the female, they come upon the vaginal surface, vulva, nymphæ, orifice of the urethra, and upon the inner aspect of the labia. They usually begin to appear in the lower part of the vagina, near its orifice, and extend towards the superior commissure. They grow with great rapidity. Even if excised with the knife or scissors, they immediately return, provided the gonorrhœa continues; and if undisturbed, they soon become large and vascular, occasioning more or less hemorrhage and severe pain when cut off. They are generally soft and spongy when situated in these parts, and constitute one of the greatest inconveniences that attend gonorrhœa in the female. In some instances, large excrescences spring from the walls of the vagina at a little distance from its orifice, and their presence will keep up a discharge for a long time after the gonorrhœa, in which they originated, has ceased. The patient, perhaps, makes no complaint; but if she engages in any active exercise, the discharge will probably return, and be as abundant as ever, and the ordinary treatment for arresting it will be employed with little or no relief.

In both sexes, vegetations collect around the verge of the anus, on the perineal integument, and within the cleft of the nates, where the natural moisture and other irritating matters are retained. In the recent state, and while lubricated with the substance exuded from the mucous surface, they are comparatively soft and white; if they remain for a considerable time, and come in contact with the air, they dry up and become quite hard, and of a dark color. Sometimes they are broad, thick and flattened; or they may have a small pedicle or stem, by which they are attached to the corium from which they germinate, and present a form not unlike a grain of wheat or rice. Their anatomical structure consists of a thick, firm investment of epithelial laminæ and newly-formed cellular tissue which is usually well supplied with blood vessels and nervous loops, and hence the pain and bleeding when growths are removed. The epithelium is not perforated, but is pushed up without being broken as the vegetation grows. I have seen them in male and female subjects, who were, and always had been, otherwise exempt from disease in the parts occupied by these morbid growths, but who had no practical notions of personal cleanliness. It is by no means difficult to believe that such individuals are just the ones to furnish the elements for the formation of these adventitious appendages. The wonder is that they do not occur more frequently.

Vegetations of a non-specific nature are now and then complicated with true condylomata, which proceed from a venereal cause, and which belong to the circle of secondary symptoms.

When these condylomatous excrescences exist, other syphilitic phenomena will be present also; or the history of the case will show that they have existed at some former period; and the physician will seldom have any difficulty in assuming the right position as regards the diagnosis. Some authorities make this distinction—that simple vegetations are always pedunculated, while those that are really syphilitic are always sessile and seated on a broad base; and the granular patch is of a dirty red or whitish hue—rather flat than prominent; secretes a watery, yellowish discharge, and having a most disgusting odor. But nothing short of a truthful history of the case can furnish a perfectly reliable basis on which to establish a correct diagnosis. Mere appearances may deceive the most practiced eye. This they always have done and always will do.

GONORRHŒAL RHEUMATISM.

Medical science has not as yet shed any light upon the specific cause of this disease. But the circumstances which appear to bring this cause, whatever it may be, into active operation in certain individuals, are for the most part within our comprehension. The practitioner usually ascertains upon inquiry, that the patient in whom the affliction is developed as a complication of urethral discharge, possessses some marked peculiarity of temperament — very probably the lymphatic; or has a hereditary tendency to rheumatism or gout; or perhaps is suffering from nervous debility or constitutional debility; or has exposed himself to some adverse agency, as cold, and wet, and wind. It is frequently associated with orchitis. It occasionally seizes upon the fleshy parts of the frame, as the shoulders, the inter-costal muscles, the hips, the thighs, soles of the feet, etc. But the most usual, and by far the most important and inveterate form which the complaint assumes, is that which is known under the designation of articular or gonorrhœal rheumatism. or gonorrhœal inflammation of the synovial membranes. Some men are sure to have articular rheumatism whenever they contract gon-

orrhœa; and it is by no means uncommon for patients who have the synovial inflammation, to have,
simultaneously, some form of ophthalmia.

This singular affection, like that which diffuses itself among the muscular and fibrous tissues as a
complication of a gonorrhœal discharge, may come
on at any period, although it seldom shows itself
until the latter has materially declined or entirely
ceased. The knee is by preference most frequently
the seat of the disorder, but other superficial articulations are liable to be attacked. The synovial
sheaths of the extensor tendons on the wrist and
instep are sometimes involved. In most instances,
only one joint is implicated at a time; in other cases
the disease invades several articulations at once.
The inflammatory action is suddenly lighted up,
and without previous warning, is not particularly
violent in its features, is wont to linger as a sub-
acute affection for an indefinite period, to the discomfort of the patient and the embarassment of the
physician. In consequence of synovial effusion, the
joint becomes much enlarged; and if the complaint
occupy the knee, the fluctuation of the effused fluid
can easily be detected at an early period.

The effusion remains for several months after the
other symtoms have disappeared.

In spite of every exertion of the medical attendant for its removal, the swelling yields with great
reluctance; and often, on slight provocations, returns
with surprising rapidity, first in one knee, then in

the other; and in this way the patient is tormented for years. There is ordinarily but little constitutional disturbance. The integument covering the joint preserves its natural temperature and color for a considerable time, even when there is a great increase in the size of the joint. In some rare instances, the accompanying symptoms become general and severe. The pulse is full and quick, the stomach and other organs of digestion sympathize, and the patient falls into a decline. In other individuals, the inflammation will proceed through its whole course without being attended with any symtoms of effusion. In still other cases, endo-carditis and effusion into the pericardium have taken place; also compression of the spinal cord and of the brain, and which appeared to follow the articular affections.

The usual symtoms of acute rheumatism are seldom developed, and when they are manifested, they are moderate in degree; the constitutional disturbance being quite trifling, when contrasted with the severity of the local arthritic affection.

Suppuration sometimes takes place, but this or the formation of abscesses within or around the joint is a rare accident.

The almost total absence of pain, the normal aspect and warmth of the skin, and the condition of the system usually attendant on the complaint in its early stages, are to be set down as the most reliable characteristic marks which it exhibits, and may serve, when taken in connection with the history of the patient, as sufficient grounds for separating it from ordinary rheumatism, and from those neuralgic and nocturnal pains which a person not unfrequently experiences in the latter stages of CONSTITUTIONAL SYPHILIS.

GONORRHŒA IN THE FEMALE.

Among what we term in medical parlance female diseases, and which we are called upon to investigate and treat; gonorrhœa proceeding from some portion of the generative system of the female, is one of the most common. The investigation of this disease, is often beset with difficulty and embarrassment. The impossibility of determining in all cases between a gonorrhœa resulting from infections, and one that has no such origin, is acknowledged by all practitioners. Such instances are occasionally met with in the male subject, but in the female they are very frequent. Especially do they occur in women who have long been troubled with some chronic secretion of obscure character, assuming different appearances at different epochs; being at one period mucous, at another mucous and pus, or mucous and blood; and so on, through still other transformations; sometimes attended with but little inconvenience, at other times fretting and irritating the surface over which it flows. To these chronic cases the difficulty of discrimination is chiefly confined.

Neither chemical nor pathological investigations

have as yet furnished anything like the requisite data by which we might decide in any given case as to the contagious or non-contagious properties of these abnormal exudations. Were we at liberty to make experiments in the inoculation of these vitiated secretions, we should still fail to have any absolute criterion, or to acquire any incontestible evidence in the premises, so far as relates to the true gonorrhœal element derived by contagion from another. For it must be admitted that the vaginal secretions of some females who are perfectly chaste and entirely free from all gonorrhœal taint, may give rise to urethral inflammation and gonorrhœa in some men. Leucorrhœa has the credit of doing this. The same power is claimed in behalf of normal menstrual fluid. There are not a few able writers who have implicit faith in the ability of both these secretions to provoke a gonorrhœal discharge.

Candor, indeed, compels me to go farther, and to admit that an acrid condition of the ordinary mucous moisture—the epithelial exudation from the uterus or the vagina—may generate a gonorrhœa in the male. But this male, in my opinion, must be endowed with some peculiar idiosyncrasy, some remarkable aptitude, which predisposes him to receive the infection. Thus, extraordinary conditions appertaining to both parties at the same time, may occasion non-specific symptoms in a man, that cannot be distinguished in their severity, duration, or complications, from those phenomena attributable to a contagion derived from a woman, who has, and who gives, a veritable gonorrhœa at the moment of sexual congress. Such instances are, however, exceedingly rare. The anatomical differences which I have observed in gonorrhœal inflammation, are the very great quantity of pus secreted, the extreme redness, congestion, and swelling of the mucous membrane, the extension of the inflammation to the urethra, and its extreme intractability to treatment.

Young female children are sometimes troubled with a diseased condition of the genital organs, presenting symptoms very much like those arising in the female of adult age. The trouble usually commencing in the prepuce of the clitoris, which from some accidental cause, becomes inflamed; and the affection afterwards extends gradually to the labia, nymphæ, and perhaps to the vagina. In some instances, small ulcerations form here and there upon the mucous membrane, which yields very little purulent discharge. In other cases, erosions takes place, or there is · an aphthous condition of the parts, attended with a serous exudation more or less copious, and irritating to the surface with which it comes in contact. In still other instances, but of very infrequent occurrence, a leucorrhœal discharge is noticed, apparently from the vagina, while the other associate organs remain healthy, and the child is otherwise well. In none of these cases do the symptoms

assume a specific character. They may awaken
alarm in the mind of the mother, and sometimes
suspicion may be excited that foul play has been
practised upon the child by a person having a
gonorrhœal or venereal affection, when such is not
the fact.

Gonorrhœal inflammation in women, attended
with a specific discharge, eminently contagious,
attacks the mucous membrane of the vulva, the
vagina, urethra and uterus. In very mild cases,
the abnormal action is confined to this membrane ;
but, in most instances, it penetrates into the subjacent tissues.

It is usually limited to some portions of the genito-urinary apparatus, although in certain cases which
have been neglected, or which, from some special
circumstances, resist the ordinary therapeutic measures, the malady propagates itself throughout all
the organs. Among the ulterior accidents resulting
from gonorrhœa, may be mentioned, cystitis, nephritis, inflammation and obliteration of the Fallopian
tubes, ovaritis, sterility, peritonitis, inflammation,
and suppuration of the inguinal lymphatic glands
and of the labia majora, chronic enlargement of the
nymphæ, &c.

INFLAMMATION OF THE VAGINA.

Vaginitis is both acute and chronic ; when originating in contagion. it begins by acute inflamma-

tion, and subsides into the chronic catarrhal form before it ceases altogether.

The disorder commences at the fore-part of the vagina. It spreads, as some suppose, by the irritation of its secretions flowing over adjacent parts, but it is also possible that this inflammation extends along the substance of the tissue in which it is seated, as an erysipelatous inflammation extends along the tissue which it has attacked. By whatever mode it extends, the gonorrhœal inflammation invades usually the vulva, the urethra, the upper part of the vagina, and the cervical portion of the uterus ; at this part it commonly passes within the meatus to the cervix. But beyond this point the inflammation seldom extends, though on rare occasions, as I have said, it may reach the substance of the uterus, or the peritoneum. &c.

Acute vaginitis may be set up by several causes, besides contact with gonorrhœal matter.

Violent sexual interconse, especially when that is much repeated about the menstrual period, often causes inflammation of the mucous membrane. Vaginitis is also commonly seen in children who have been subjected to criminal attacks, and it may occur in newly married women. The presence of foreign bodies, such as a sponge, or pessary, or strong injection, when used for some disease of the uterus, will cause vaginitis.

The acute vaginitis of contagion is more violent than vaginitis non-specific.

A few days after coitus, a ˙ tickling sensation, changing to heat and burning, occupies the external genitals. The mucous membrane grows dry, brightly red, and tender, the labia swell, and cause discomfort or pain in walking. Sometimes even sitting down must be cautiously done to avoid pain ; scalding with micturition is usual.

The swelling often becomes considerable by the oedema extending throughout the external genitals; a condition which corresponds to balanitis in the male is thus produced.

Dull aching pain in the sacral region, and in the limbs or body generally, is not infrequent when the attack is severe. The discharge is at first thin and watery, and small in quantity ; but it soon grows whitish-yellow, or even greenish in color, of an offensive odor, and so profuse that it flows copiously from the vagina when that is opened by the finger. If the finger is passed into the vagina, the papillæ are felt to be prominent and distinct on the forepart of the mucous membrane. When the speculum can be introduced, the mucous membrane of the whole vagina, and often over the vaginal portion of the uterus, is seen to be bright red, while around the os tincæ, it may be raised into a group of papillæ,—which give the cervix a strawberry-like appearance. These papillæ or granulations are sometimes ulcerated, and then form yellowish dots about the margin of the os uteri. The cul de sac behind the neck of the uterus is generally filled with

thick yellow matter, and the epithelium of the whole
of the vagina is easily abraded, so that it bleeds if
any roughness is employed in using the speculum.
When the inflammation is very intense, the constitution participates in the disturbance.

There is loss of appetite, thirst, hot skin, pains in
the limbs and restlessness, with other signs of
fever.

When the acute congestion and copious discharge
have continued a few days the irritation subsides,
the discharge is whiter, the mucous membrane assumes a somewhat livid hue and is very lax ; here
and there, patches of it are excoriated or even ulcerated. The granular condition is still present,
and generally very distinct. If the patient avoids
fresh irritation, the discharge gradually gets less in
quantity and more like the natural secretion. But
the inflammation often changes its ground to the
urethra, or neck of the uterus ; or it may still hang
about the upper part of the vagina, when it has
ceased near the entry. The glands of the groin
often swell and grow tender while the vaginitis is
at its height ; or the irritation may even proceed to
abscess, which is simply sympathetic and never
virulent. This complication is much more frequent
when the vulva as well as the vagina is inflamed.
There is another variety of vaginitis, called granular
vaginitis, which was at one time supposed to be peculiar and distinct from ordinary vaginitis, but is
simply the result of the congestion of the mucous

membrane being greater in certain parts than in others. It is most usually seen in pregnant women, especially when they are about twenty-eight to thirty-eight years of age. If this condition is produced, the mucous membrane is dark purplish in patches, and dotted with little granular elevations of a darker hue than the surface they spring from. The cervix uteri is very often the seat of these little granulations, and as before said, will give that part a strawberry-like appearance. ` Granular vaginitis has the same course as the ordinary vaginitis. but is a sign of obstinacy in the inflammation.

When vaginitis becomes chronic, the discharge is generally whitish, milky, even creamy, or translucent like gum, and the congestion very slight ; the reaction is always acid. The discharge consists of pavement epithelium, pus, and mucous corpuscles, and very often ·infusoriæ.

VULVITIS.

The earliest and most constant complication of gonorrhœa in women is inflammation of the external organs of generation, the larger and smaller labia, and the clitoris ; this is called vulvitis, and is the analogue of balano-posthitis in the male. The causes are irritation of all kinds ; habitual neglect of cleanliness, especially if the patient is fat, and the weather warm, will cause inflammation without any gonorrhœal contagion. But this is the most frequent cause of vulvitis, either by the inflammation extending from the vagina to the vulva, or less frequently the disorder begins there and spreads to the vagina. An inflamed chancre and violent masturbation are occasionally causes of vulvitis when gonorrhœa is not present.

The symptoms begin with itching, smarting, redness, and swelling of the large and small labia, from which the redness generally extends to the skin of the perineum and thighs. The secretion of the sebaceous glands is greatly increased, and often collects in thick adherent layers in the folds of the mucous membrane. An offensive muco-purulent discharge drains from the vulva, which frequently causes erythema, erosions, and inflammation of the hair follicles of the skin outside.

If this secretion is wiped off, the glandulæ project in small, round, yellowish eminences on the red surface. While the parts are swollen, walking and even sitting upright are very painful. When the irritation is great, or in weakly persons, the inflammation becomes often erysipelatous, and then it may cause abscess and sloughing of the labia and parts adjacent. The abscesses generally arise from suppuration in the sebaceous glands, or in the glands of Bartholine, and they greatly enhance the severity of the disorder. Like vaginitis, vulvitis occasionally excites sympathetic irritation of the inguinal lymphatic glands and bubo.

URETHRITIS.

This is a very frequent accompaniment of gonorrhœal vaginitis, but is extremely rare as a simple disorder. The symptoms vary much, according to the intensity of the neighboring inflammation in the vagina or vulva. When the urethritis is very acute, the patient complains of smarting and frequent desire to make water, but unless this is the case she generally does not complain of anything more than a little itching at the meatus ; tenesmus, or even increase of pain in making water, is rarely acknowledged by the patient. Cystitis is comparatively unknown. The mucous membrane is red and swollen around the meatus ; the redness being often punctiform, and the papilla between the meatus urinarius and vagina is thrust prominently forward.

There is generally a whitish muco-purulent or purulent discharge oozing from the meatus, though when the inflammation has become chronic it often needs some trouble to make the existence of the discharge evident. When the patient has recently passed water, the urethra may be quite clear of discharge. In such cases the ducts of the follicles which open at the surface close to the meatus urinarius, some outside it, will exude matter that is the remains of a gonorrhœal inflammation, which has spread along them as well as into the urethra.

Urethritis continues in the chronic stage an indefinite time, and as it takes origin in contagion,

it is impossible to say when it ceases to be dangerous and unable to excite gonorrhœa in others.

ACUTE INFLAMMATION OF THE CERVIX AND OS UTERI.

When vaginitis reaches the fundus, it very commonly extends over the vaginal part of the uterus,
and enters the os, by which it may attain the cavity
of the uterus, but the inflammation is usually confined to the cervix.

The symptoms are generally combined with those
of vaginitis ; but the irritation of the uterus is de-
noted generally by a sudden accession of constitutional disturbance, a chill, or even a shiver, loss of
appetite, or nausea.

When these are well marked, the cavity of the
uterus is involved as well as the neck.

If pain at the sacrum has accompanied the vaginitis, it increases, and, if not present before this
symptom, is rarely absent when inflammation of the
cervix begins.   There often is also pain at the hypo-
gastrium, and dragging sensation of the groins.
The uterus is sometimes tender when pressed, but
not enlarged.

Irritation of the bladder and rectum produces
frequent desire to urinate and tenesmus, and the
urine is turbid with lithates.   By the fourth or fifth
day the constitutional disturbance ceases, and a discharge appears, at first clear, then opaque, making
stiff spots on the linen.   The secretion from the
neck of the uterus has much greater viscidity than

the vaginal pus, but when mixed with that coming from the cavity of the uterus, assumes a creamy appearance, little distinguishable from the pus secreted in the vagina.

It differs from the latter, however, in being alkaline, and does not produce eczema or irritation of the skin over which it may flow. The cervix uteri when examined, is seen to be swollen, red, and excoriated round the os. which is dilated and filled with discharge.

This discharge varies very much with the stage of the disorder ; while the cervix is swollen and red, the discharge is very tenacious and copious, and is extremely difficult to extract from the cervix. "This is the early stage of acute congestion. But in a few days the redness of the cervix lessens, the swelling also is less, and the discharge, which has become purulent, trickles freely from the os uteri, especially if the patient is told to bear down for a moment. This is the stage of acute suppuration ; and when the discharge is copious or escapes from the os in gushes, it is furnished by the interior of the uterus as well as by the neck. If the uterus is examined it will be found large and tender. In a week, or sometimes less, the discharge will be again different. In this third stage it is much less in quantity, more viscid than when in the second stage, but still purulent. The os is often superficially ulcerated, and if the discharge be cleared away, the cervix within is seen to be excoriated also.

The uterus is no longer tender, but the cervix is hard and enlarged, sometimes very considerably, when the chronic congestion has continued a long time.

The inflammation has now reached the stage of chronic uterine catarrh, and is not distinguishable from a catarrh produced by other causes than gonorrhœal inflammation. If the inflammation does not lapse into a chronic catarrh, the redness and swelling depart, the sensation of fulness and irritation in the pelvic organ ceases, and the discharge, becoming serous, rapidly diminishes.

There is very little peculiarity about inflammation of the cervix uteri when originating in gonorrhœal vaginitis that distinguishes it from inflammation through other causes. Yet there can be no doubt that a discharge of this kind is constantly the cause of gonorrhœa in men, and the more so, because in its chronic form it often escapes the patient's attention altogether. The discharge, in all probability, arises from contagion, if there has recently been vaginitis, or if any discharge can be obtained from the urethra.

But when there is no urethral discharge, no vaginitis, and the inflammation set in during or shortly after the menstrual period ; if the patient has been exposed to cold, fatigue, or is newly married, the disorder has probably arisen independently of gonorrhœal contagion.

METRITIS.

Inflammation of the substance of the womb is described by certain authors as a consequence of gonorrhœa. If it really occurs this complication is excessively rare, and has nothing distinctive from metritis through other causes.

Its symptoms are very much those which accompany catarrhal inflammation of the interior of the uterus, beginning with shivering, loss of appetite, pain and fulness in the pelvis, with irritation of the rectum.

If the uterus is examined, the fundus is enlarged, and tender when touched.

SYPHILIS.

The origin and history of this dreadful disease are enveloped in so much mystery and obscurity that it is probably impossible to tell when and where it was first known, and spoken of as a separate and distinct disease. It doubtless existed in some parts of the old world—in Asia, Africa, and it may be in Eastern Europe—as far back at least as the earliest records of history extend, and most likely in all ages of the world, since it has been inhabited by man. Chinese medical literature affords evidence of the existence of syphilis in that country, and of its treatment many centuries before the birth of Christ, and we know that the Bible contains evidence of a similar disease among the Jews and the surrounding heathen nations, as far back as the days of Moses,

and the earlier history of the Jewish tribes. Who
knows but the leprosy, so often spoken of in the Old
Testament, and also in the New, was one form of
syphilis? It is the opinion of some of the best writers on medicine and the history of certain diseases,
that the leprosy of the Old Testament was but the
constitutional or secondary form of syphilis, and I
am inclined to the same opinion. As early as the
middle of the fifteenth century it is known that laws
were made in England and France to regulate
"houses of ill-fame" or brothels, so as to prevent
the spread of venereal diseases, both syphilis and
gonorrhœa being probably regarded then as one and
the same disease ; for it is well known that physicians and medical writers contended long since then
that these two diseases were but different forms of
the same disease.

The constitutional or secondary form seems not
to have been known, or if known, was not properly
recognized and understood. In 1495 it occurred as
an epidemic in Naples among the French and Ital-
ian armies, creating the greatest alarm, and causing the impression that it was a new disease.
Hence the origin of the fact that there are two syphilitic diseases—chancroid and syphilis proper.
It was called the "French disease," because it was
thought to have been brought to Naples by the
French army, at that time, and the extreme viru-
lence and terrible violence with which it prevailed,
gave rise to the other erroneous assumption that it

was a new disease, or a separate and distinct one from that which had before been known as chancre and bubo, instead of the same disease in a more aggravated form, as it really was. There are, properly speaking, but two venereal diseases, that is diseases of the genital organs, communicated by coitus, or sexual intercourse, and these are gonorhœa and syphilis. Gonorrhœa is simply a local, inflammatory disease, commonly called clap. Syphilis embraces what is known as chancre and chancroid, bubo, and the attending sequelæ, but constituting one disease.

We may consider the fact as established beyond reasonable doubt, that in all the varieties of the disease, there is but one true poison of syphilis, which poison produces different effects, according to the nature of the tissue and the peculiar idiosyncrasy of the constitution, in which the disease is manifested; all these different phenomena depending on the same morbific cause.

The causes of syphilis are predisposing and exciting. Predisposing causes are conditions facilitating the spread or increasing the severity of the disease. Thus, it is more severe in cold than in temperate climates; and in hot ones for natives of cooler climates. Any cause which enfeebles the constitution of the individual increases the severity of the disease, among which are starvation, drunkenness, &c. All races are subject to the disease; when it invades the district not previously accustomed to it, its course, like that of other contagious diseases, becomes for a time severe. Probably individuals exist who are insusceptible to syphilis, and escape contagion of that disease, as they escape contagion of small-pox, &c. .

The sole exciting cause of syphilis is a subtle principle called the virus. It must be passed from the infected to the non-infected.

Of the essence—the intrinsic nature—of the microscopic forms of this virus or animal poison, we know nothing. As yet it has proved too subtle for detection. Whatever it may be, in any stage of its vitality, it remains shrouded in the same darkness that conceals from our comprehension the elementary nature of the variolous substance, or the morbific principle of hydrophobia, typhus fever, or cholera.

The poison almost always enters at a breach of surface. Experience is generally against its absorption through unabraded surfaces.

The vehicles of the virus are: the secretions of all early syphilitic eruptions and the blood, but they usually cease to be contagious when the disease is almost extinct, and only the so-called tertiary affections are left.

The secretions of co-existing diseases in syphilitic persons may be also contagious.

Close contact between individuals is eminently favorable, though not necessary, for communicating the disease; hence sexual intercouse, kissing, and suckling, are the usual modes of immediate contagion; while passing of spoons, cups, or any such thing from mouth to mouth, and vaccination are modes of mediate contagion.

There is probably no appreciable interval between the application of the virus to a denuded surface and its absorption; hence washing or cauterizations, after contagion, in the hope of preventing the disease, are useless, because the mischief they should prevent is already done.

In respect to contagion by inheritance our knowledge is imperfect, concerning the ways in which constitutional syphilis is transmitted from parent to child.

There is no doubt that if the mother is infected before or at conception, the child is very likely to receive the disease.

Probably the child may contract the disease, if the mother is infected in the early months of pregnancy. If she is infected after the seventh month, the child often escapes.

As the disease subsides in the mother, the chances of escape for the child greatly increase, and after the second or third year, the child commonly escapes.

The child may receive the disease from the father.

It is believed, also, that the child may inherit the disease from the father, while the mother escapes; but this is not yet established.

INCUBATION.

After inoculation, the virus of syphilis sometimes remains latent, giving no signs of its presence for a length of time, while at other times it begins to act almost immediately.

The time from the contact of the virus till its first perceptible effect is called the period of incubation.

This interval between impure connection, and the manifestation of local symptoms varies considerably, according to the condition and anatomical structure of the part in which the virus is deposited. If this spot happen to be denuded of its cuticular or epithelial covering, inoculation will show itself, without doubt, and at an earlier moment than it would if there were no such abrasion. It is probable, also, that the specific appearances may be developed more rapidly on the warm, moist surface of the mucous tissue than on the external surface. Indeed, it is very difficult to inoculate through the sound skin .

So as the circumstances of inoculation vary, the time between exposure and the supervention of morbid phenomena or inoculation varies.

It varies from twenty-four hours to ninety days.

Syphilis is usually divided into three stages, and each has symptoms peculiar to itself. These are known as Primary, Secondary and Tertiary.

PRIMARY STAGE.

The lesions peculiar to primary syphilis are the chancre or ulcer, and an enlargement of the lymphatic glands of the groin or bubo.

INITIAL MANIFESTATIONS OF SYPHILIS, CHANCRE,

The size, appearance and shape of the chancre differ widely in various cases, being influenced to a considerable degree by its location and circumstances. They also differ in degree of development, and in diversity of structure.

Although a chancre may occur on any part of the body, yet it is by far most common on the genital organs. Its most common sites are the head of the penis and prepuce, the vulva, vagina and uterus. The disease may also attack the urethra in both sexes, especially in the male, although the occurrence is uncommon. Any portion of the head and fore-skin of the penis may be affected, but of the former the corona, or rather the fossa, just behind corona, and the surface on each side of the frænum are most liable to be involved from the circumstance that these parts are particularly apt to retain the infecting matter; for the same reason the free extremity of the prepuce is very prone to suffer. A severe chancre occasionally forms on the body or root of the penis. In the female the disease sometimes occurs on the perinæum, on the outer surface of the labium, and around the anus.

There are six different kinds of chancres: 1, *The elevated desquamating* chancre; 2, the *superficial* chancre; 3, the *indolent* chancre, with a hard base; 4, the *masked* chancre; 5, the *inflammatory* chancre; 6, the *phagedenic* chancre. .

1. The *desquamating* chancre begins by forming a small solid elevation at the point of inoculation; this, at first the size of a pin's head, extends until it may reach that of a sixpence or a shilling. The skin around retains its natural aspect, and no inconvenience, except now and then a little itching, is ·felt. The color is reddish-coppery, or reddish-purple, like raw ham. The surface, slightly raised above the skin, is flat and smooth, being covered by a few thin scales or dry epithelium. Not unfrequently, the papulæ undergoes no further change, but after five or six weeks grows pale and subsides, leaving no trace of its presence.

When the site of inoculation is the scar of a previous chancre, the cicatrix is thickened by this new deposit, which then frequently assumes an irregular form; instead of round or oval, it becomes angular, or linear; in these cases the coppery tint is often altogether absent, and the surface retains then the same hue as that of the surrounding skin.

This form is most common on the skin in situations which are kept dry and not chafed.

2. The *superficial* chancre comes between the dry scaling sore and the well-marked ulcer; common localities for it are under the surface of the foreskin,

or in women the opposed surfaces of the nymphæ, where the parts are constantly moist. For its
production the surface of the elevated papulæ becomes red, secretes a plentiful fluid, usually thin
and serous, but occasionally puriform.

These eroded surfaces are similar in appearance
to the mucous patches of the general eruption,
which like these owe their character entirely to the
constant moisture.

Sometimes, on the skin or sheath of the penis the
induration is very scanty, the surface consequently
is only slightly raised; and it usually secretes a little
viscid discharge, but has no tendency to extend, nor,
unless irritated by dirt, to suppurate.

Its edges are clearly defined, which peculiarity
with the absence of induration, causes it to slightly
resemble the inflamed chancre.

3. The *indolent* chancre with a hard base, or indurated chancre begins exactly in the same manner
as the desquamating sore; but the surface, instead
of stopping short at desquamation, ulcerates. The
ulceration begins at the centre and spreads outwards through the indurated papulæ, but does not
extend beyond the papulæ, whence the cicatrix or
scar is very small when the ulcer heals, and is often
imperceptible.

The base of the sore is hard and resisting, feeling
between the finger and thumb like a cup of gristle
set in the skin; its surface is covered by a scanty ad-
hesive yellow discharge, the edges are sloping,

rounded, and the induration extends a little beyond the extent of the ulcer. The progress is always slow, and, if the sore is kept clean and free from irritation, terminates by cessation of the ulceration, cicatrization of the surface, and absorption of the indurated deposit.

4. When a chancre is situated in the urethra, in the vagina, or upon the os tincæ, it is called the concealed or *masked* chancre.

It is this sore upon which supervene, sooner or later, these consecutive symptoms that were formerly supposed to have their origin in gonorrhœa; and hence the latter affection was believed to be a genuine syphilitic malady by some medical practitioners.

This sore may exist at any point of the urethral canal, between the external orifice and the bladder.

The most frequent site, however, is just within the meatus. The discharge does not appear till a late day after suspicious connection, when it is intermittent, and occurs at irregular intervals, and is variable in character, being sometimes thin, scanty, and sanious, and at other times thick and profuse, or presenting a tenacious slough, similar to what is cast off from the indurated chancre in its ulcerative stage.

The presence of a distinct induration at the spot where the chancre is concealed, may be felt on pressure with the finger; except where it is deep seated, and then the diagnosis becomes very difficult.

Varieties of this chancre and its situation sometimes give rise to very serious mutilations. If it
be at the orifice of the urethra, it may occasion contraction of that portion of the canal, so as to require the long-continued use of small bougies to prevent closure of the mouth.

Sometimes when the chancre is seated at a distance from the entrance of the canal, it causes, on
healing, a troublesome traumatic stricture, which is
by no means easily cured. In other instances the
ulcerative process extends through the entire parts,
and perforations take place, usually immediately behind the glan-penis; and large portions even of the
urethra and of the bladder, are destroyed, the patient dying in consequence.

5. *Inflammatory* chancre is the simple venereal
sore, assuming an inflammatory character, and the
latter condition may manifest itself at any period of
the accident.

Sometimes the pain, swelling, and other concomitant symptoms arise very suddenly; and increase
with great rapidity; and, if not arrested, gangrene
and sloughing will take place speedily.

Where a careful and judicious line of treatment
is adopted, this form of chancre is seldom seen.
The state of things implied by the term inflammatory chancre is generally induced in consequence of
some irritating or caustic substance applied to the
sore, in the haste to destroy it. Patients of irregular
habits, and of sanguineous temperament are more

commonly susceptible to this variety of chancre.

Sometimes gangrene and sloughing may be so destructive as to compel, as a last resort, the operation for amputation of the penis.

6. The *phagedenic* chancre is the result generally of acute inflammation unsuccessfully treated. Inflammatory chancre is liable to progress to a state of gangrene and sloughing, and the phagedenic sore is the ultimate stage or point to which inflam- . mation can extend.

The phagedenic chancre always denotes a de-praved condition of the animal economy. The patient looks haggard, has what we call a broken-down constitution, induced perhaps, by a variety of causes—such as intemperate habits, excessive de-bauchery, and other irregularities connected with a life of dissipation, confinement in the wards of a badly ventilated hospital, or living in any unwhole-some situation, and any other adverse conditions.

Sailors who have been engaged in long service, and who consequently have been exposed to the hard vicissitudes of the sea, and individuals of a scrofulous and lymphatic diathesis and flabby mus-cular fibre, are also some of those in whom phaged-enic chancre is apt to appear.

The progress of this chancre, if neglected, is very rapid; the constitutional symptoms, to which it gives rise, are of a more serious type than those at-tending any other primary sore. Sometimes, when the phagedena seizes upon the prepuce, the whole of this membrane will be swept away in thirty hours; and where the glans is attacked, the destructive action advances with nearly equal rapidity, involving all the structures of the organ, which in two or three days becomes a revolting mass of putridity.

INFLAMMATION OF THE LYMPHATIC GLANDS OR BUBO.

The enlargement of the glands takes place in two ways. The first and more common variety, called sympathetic bubo, is simply an inflammation of the lymphatic glands and their surrounding cellular tissue from the irritation of the chancre. This bubo may occur at any time during the progress of a chancre, though most frequently in the first two weeks. The gland which first receives the lymphatics, swells and grows very tender, rendering walking, and even standing, painful. In the early stage it can be distinctly felt under the skin, but soon it is masked by congestion and inflammation of the cellular·tissue surrounding it, and thus forms an oval tumor lying over Poupart's ligament. The skin over the swelling assumes a dusky red tint, and grows soft and doughy to the touch. Pus forms in the congested cellular tissue around the gland, and presently the abscess bursts through the skin, its contents escape, and the cavity heals by granulation in the ordinary way. The duration of the bubo in this case will be a month or six weeks, but it is often prolonged by the obstinate sinuses which are left under the skin.

In one form, called the phlegmonous bubo, the enlargement is much slower; the whole group of glands are attacked, and produce a doughy, ill-defined, somewhat tender swelling, in which the separate glands cannot be distinguished from each other. The skin after some week's chronic congestion, becomes a dark, reddish-purple. In course of time, fluctuation can be detected at several points, from suppuration beginning at the same time, in different parts of the cellular tissue. The pus thus formed makes its way to the surface, and tunnels several sinuses, which last many months before they heal. This variety of bubo has been also called scrofulous bubo, from its occurring in scrofulous persons, and from resembling other scrofulous lymphatic abscesses.

Abscesses of this kind usually extend outwards towards the iliac spine, as well as towards the perineum. Their duration much depends on the patient's general health, and kind of treatment pursued.

When the bubo is healed, it leaves a small shrunken cicatrix, at first dark in color, but subsequently turning white.

Another form of bubo is where suppuration is excited in the gland itself by the contagious matter being conveyed directly from the chancre along the absorbents. The inflammatory action inside the gland quickly extends to the cellular tissue, forming an abscess around the gland, which is inoculated by the absorbed contagious matter that is set free when the gland breaks up or is punctured. The abscess thus itself becomes a chancre, and resembles the original sore in all its characters, though much exceeding it in size.

In its course this bubo, virulent bubo, is very similar to the sympathetic bubo. It is not so frequent as the former, and it is uncertain in the time of its appearance; its duration is commonly a few weeks, but it may last much longer.

Usually one gland only is attacked, and that acutely. There is considerable pain in the part, and general disturbance. When the abscess is opeこed and inoculated with the matter within the gland, the surface becomes irregular and worm-eaten; the borders hardened, eroded, and often much undermined; the undermined skin grows dull violet in color, now and then an isolated bit sloughs off; the discharge is puriform, plentiful, thinner than that of the original abscess, but contagious and inoculable on the patient himself.

The abscess, thus converted into a very large chancre, may become phagedenic and serpiginous, and before it heals may spread over a wide surface, and cause considerable loss of tissue.

The fascia is sometimes laid bare in the floor of of the ulcer, and the other lymphatic glands lying on it are exposed.

The veins around may ulcerate and be trouble-some, even dangerous hemorrhage occurs, or a great part of the skin of the groin, thigh, or abdomen, may be destroyed. The duration is ordinarily three to four months, but sometimes it may last for one or two years.

Bubo without chancre was supposed to result from the venereal matter entering a breach of sur-face and passing along the lymphatics to the gland, there causing inflammation without producing a sore at the point of contagion. But this is a mis-take. They are not the result of venereal poison, but one of the sequences of venery.

They occur generally in young, weakly persons, and invariably cause a good deal of constitutional disturbance. They are caused by the fatigue of vio-lent intercourse, just as severe exercise in walking, or running, will produce an abscess of the lympha-tics, and under proper treatment quickly heal. They are never the premonitory signs of general syphilitic eruptions.

Besides the foregoing varieties of irritation and inflammation of the lymphatic glands, the lympha-tic vessels leading to the glands are themselves sometimes inflamed, if the sore be placed on the prepuce or skin of the penis. The symptoms are a ridgy swelling, like a knotty string, on the back of the penis, tender and often red; this lasts ten or fourteen days, and then subsides.

Occasionally little abscesses form along the inflamed vessel, which become ulcers or chancres, and which are very tedious, as they leave sinuses that fill and break alternately, with little tendency to heal if left to themselves.

SECONDARY STAGE.

This stage consists in the appearance of eruptions upon the skin, and ulcers upon mucous membranes in various parts of the body.

This period begins about ten weeks after contagion, six or seven after induration of the point of inoculation, and four or five after the lymphatic glands begin to enlarge.

Malaise and pyrexia precede or accompany the outbreak of the rash. At this time the temperature of the body is sometimes a little raised. The febrile action and pain may even be intense, and the former has been known to assume a periodic intermitting course. The fever subsides when the eruption is fully out.

The eruptions resemble many of the ordinary cutaneous eruptions; hence, the various forms have been named accordingly. They are distinguished from the latter, however, by characters they have in common, and by some peculiar to each.

The papular rash generally forms the base on which the syphilitic scaling, pustular and suppurating rashes develop. In the early stages both sides of the body, both arms, both legs, may be beset with spots, because the virus producing pervades all parts of the body. The color at first is often bright red, but it changes quickly to the hue of raw ham or assumes a coppery tint. As the eruption fades, the brown color becomes more distinct, and ultimately turns to brownish-gray before disappearing altogether.

Syphilitic rashes are almost always free from heat, itching or smarting, which symptoms are a common character of most non-syphilitic affections of the skin, and often their most prominent symptom.

The most favorite localities chosen by the eruption are the trunk, the forehead, especially along the border of the scalp, the margins of the nostrils, and the nape of the neck. The outer aspects of the extremities more often escape, and the backs of the hands and feet are rarely marked.

When the disease is losing its activity, the eruptions which then appear are seldom spread widely over the body. Their brown tint is well marked.

They are prone to ulcerate, slow in progress, and the ulcers leave indelible scars.

The rashes peculiar to syphilis are divided into five general classes, as follows: *macular* and *papular* eruptions, *vesicular* and *pustular*, and *tubercular;* of which the first is by far the most common.

1. *Macular eruptions:* Roseola is about the only important rash in this division. It is the earliest rash after infection, probably always present though often overlooked. It consists of spots, rosy-red and fading under pressure at first, then coppery brown,

usually slightly elevated, sometimes desquamating as the rash subsides. The flanks and chest are the common seat of the eruption, but in rare cases it spreads all over the body, head and limbs.

2. *Papular eruptions:* In this class there are many subdivisions, according to the size and arrangement of the papules. When they are minute they are called *miliaria*, or *lichen;* when small, *lenticularis;* when large, desquamating, and irregularly scattered, *psoriasis;* when arranged into groups of circles or figures of eight, *syphilitic lepra;* when on the palm and soles, *psoriasis palmaris;* when altered by exposure to continual moisture, *mucous patches; lichen* and *lenticularis* are most frequent in the first six months after contagion; *psoriasis* comes rather later; *syphilitic lepra* and *psoriasis palmaris* are most often seen when the disease is of long standing; *mucous patches* are met with both early and late in the disease. The papules attack all parts of the body, and are the eruptions which most frequently relapse; in this way they often succeed other forms. The structure of the papule consists in a solid elevation of the skin, which commonly begins in a hair or sebaceous follicle, that grows in a less or greater degree in the smaller or larger papules. The color common to all papular eruptions is bright rosy at first, then fading to coppery or purplish brown. When the papule reaches full development, the cuticle separates in dry scales. The usual accompaniments of these eruptions are pains in the

bones, fall of the hair, iritis, ulcerated papules on the fauces, and enlarged lymphatic glands on various parts of the body. Moist papular eruptions form at the outlets of the body generally, or where they are kept moist; they assume a brighter red, and secrete a thin purulent fluid. They form flat smooth elevations, inclining to circular; when near to each other they coalesce into larger patches. If the patches are kept clean and free from irritation, they soon sink down into dry scaling surfaces. They are most frequent about the anus and the mouth. In women, mucous patches on the vulva are often the earliest and sometimes the only symptoms of syphilis which attract the patient's attention. The discharge of mucous patches is highly contagious.

When developed around the anus, they are often subdivided by fissures.

Vesicular and Pustular eruptions: These have no essential difference between them; the vesicular forms are more often seen in the earlier than in the later stages of the disease. Both are observed in febrile rather than in robust persons. They possess in common a vesicle, varying in size between a pin's head and a bean, forming the summit of an elevated areola.

After one or two days the vesicle shrinks, leaving a small scale on the areola, which falls and leaves a coppery-red papule. Sometimes, instead of drying up, the liquid becomes purulent, and the congestion of the areola increases, converting the vesicle into a pustule.

The eruptions appear usually during the first six months after infection, their course is marked by fresh crops of vesicles succeeding each other while the eruption continues; each vesicle and papule lasts about three weeks, the eruption three or four months. If the patient is well treated, the serious effect will not be produced; if he is not, very deep ulcers often form where the pustules began. This class of eruptions is also divided into others, according to their character.

Eczema is where a group of vesicles spread over a red areola. *Herpes* where the vesicles group in rings and serpentine lines, leaving the skin inside the lines unaffected.

Acne where the vesicle is filled with puriform fluid, and is developed on an elevated base.

Ecthyma, an exaggerated variety of acne, met with in very debilitated patients. It occurs on the lower limbs chiefly.

Rupia, another form which usually occurs very late in the disease. Large pustules form which soon shrink; the contents dry into a crust, the skin ulcerates under the crust, extending beneath, and forming a brownish-green hue.

Tubercular eruptions: These consist in solid, rounded elevations of the skin and subcutaneous cellular tissue. They are late affections, and appear usually in persons long infected.

There are two kinds, superficial and deep. The superficial are prominent nodules, the size of a pea, coppery or purple-brown in color, collected commonly into groups, most frequent on the face, but occurring on any part of the body; this eruption is never widely spread. The tubercles are very liable to ulcerate and then leave indelible white scars. The course is slow, for fresh tubercles appear as the old ones subside, and the eruption recurs again and again.

The deep tubercles are known as subcutaneous gummy tumors, and are much rarer than the last; they are met with only in cases of long-standing syphilis. Solid nodules form beneath the skin; presently the skin becomes absorbed over them, and bluish-red in color, they reach the surface by slow ulceration. The contents then escape, and a round swelling with a ragged ulcerated interior is left, ending in depressed white scars.

Sometimes they are reabsorbed before ulceration is reached, when they leave no trace. They are found most often on the neck, but occur on any part of the surface; they are identical with the gummy tumors of internal organs.

During this secondary stage or period of eruptions, the hair and nails often become afflicted. The hair becomes dry and withered at the outset or during the course of the cutaneous eruptions. It often falls partially from the scalp; the eyebrows, lashes and down of the body occasionally fall, too, and complete baldness is reached. But in the course of a few months under treatment the hair becomes restored.

The pustular eruptions which beset the scalp sometimes loosen the hair; it then comes away in patches, and produces bald spots. This affection is called *alopecia*.

The nails are attacked in three ways. 1st. The matrix, while a scaling rash is present elsewhere, is beset with papules; these ulcerate and destroy the nutrition of the nail, which, acting like a foreign body, causes obstinate ulcers. 2nd. The nutrition of the nail is altered, it becomes brittle, and its edge notched and ragged. 3rd. The superficial layers of the nail split or peel off, so that the nail becomes spotted and opaque at places where it is breaking away. This affection is named *onychia*.

Besides these affections during this stage others frequently happen.

Excoriations and fissures along the borders and tip of the tongue sometimes appear. Ulcers both superficial and deep form in the fauces, and attack its surface, forming most particularly on the soft palate and tonsils. These ulcerations sometimes migrate over the whole surface of the palate and pharynx. Inflammation of the lining membrane of the nose commences in this stage, with ulceration, *ozœna*, and the production of a fetid discharge that is very obstinate.

TERTIARY STAGE.

The textures which are particularly attacked in this period of the disease are the bones and internal organs of the body. In the bones, inflammation may attack either the medullary membranes or the structure itself. Where the disease is deep-seated a morbid deposit takes place, accompanied with intense suffering.

Sometimes irregularities of the bone and periosteal enlargements, termed *nodes*, reveal themselves; they are ushered in by pretty severe and constant pain. These exostoses or nodes may arise from the inner surface of the cranium, producing compression of the brain, and more or less cerebral distress, together with excessive neuralgia, partial paralysis and other serious consequences.

In the internal organs, and in the substance of the skin, gummy tumors form.

They are hard, slightly elastic, and sometimes attain the size of a hen's egg. They will lie dormant for many months or years, until inflammatory action is excited; then they form adhesions, and by slow degrees become disorganized, resulting in a peculiar kind of ulcer. Parts around undergo a gradual absorption, and a large, deep sloughing ulcer is ultimately established. They attack the skin, heart, lungs, liver, spleen, and nearly every organ of the body, and they constitute the most dangerous, tardy, and troublesome affections entailed upon the system.

SYPHILIS IN WOMEN.

In the secondary and tertiary stages of syphilis, the course of the disease is about the same as that in men. So it will not need any further description than what has already been given.

In the primary stage the symptoms are somewhat different, from the difference existing between the parts. Chancres in women are wont to assume a more unfavorable disposition than in men. These lesions may exist on the nymphæ, or on the inner surface of the labia, for a long period, and yet the patient be unsuspicious of their nature. In fact, they give little or no pain or irritation, until they acquire a large size, and the woman is hardly conscious of their presence. The first symptom that attracts her attention is a sensation of smarting and pricking, occasioned by the act of micturition. If, however, the chancres are allowed to have their own way, unchecked, they sometimes penetrate into the cellular tissue, and degenerate into sloughing ulcers, and total destruction of the parts is the result.

Females in whom this description of ulcer is found, are usually of a most abandoned character, of dissolute habits, and broken down constitution.

The sore generally commences as an abrasion, or perhaps as an angry-looking pimple, on the labia, and is soon encircled by an unhealthy, lurid areola, and from inattention, as well as in consequence of a vitiated condition of the system, it does not take on a normal granulating action, but shows a tendency

to spread in every direction, and yields a thin, serous, fœtid discharge, mixed with *debris*. At a later
period, dark-colored sloughs begin to form in quick
succession, and become more and more extensive,
until the vagina and the perineal and anal regions
are involved.

Sometimes the entire lower opening of the pelvis
is deprived of the soft parts in consequence of the
sloughing process. Excessive local pain at length
becomes a prominent and abiding symptom ; there
is high irritation or inflammatory fever, which ultimately assumes a typhoid character, with more or
less delirium; the pulse is rapid, and indicative of
great constitutional debility; the appetite fails; all
the vital functions are deranged; exhausting hemor-
rhages take place from different points of the immense ulcerated surface, and the frail victim dies
from the combined effects of bad liquor, debauchery,
and syphilis.

Fortunately this form of veneral affection is rarely
met with. But whatever form of the disease it
happens to be, the chances of cure become exceedingly small if delayed any length of time.

PROSTATITIS.

In this disease the Gland becomes painful and
swollen, and may so strongly press the neck of the
bladder as to impede or prevent the evacuation of
the organ. The disease is of comparatively rare oc-
curance in young and middle-aged persons, though
common to those of an advanced age.

The acute form generally results from an improperly treated urethral gonorrhœa, and is the most frequent cause, though it may happen from violence in using sounds, catheters, and other instruments; from the application of caustics to this part of the urethra; from immoderate coitus; from strictures, alcoholic stimulents, and exposures to cold and wet. Symptoms are: weight and dull pain in the perineum; frequent desires to urinate; some scalding sensation in deep part of urethra while urinating; bowels generally constipated and defacation attended with pain; general febrile action.

T he chronic form generally results from excessive sexual indulgence, self-abuse and sedentary habits; less frequently from gonorrhœa. Symptoms are: discharge of mucous from urethra; frequent desire to urinate; last drops dribbling away. Pain in the perineum; bowels constipated; great irritation about anus and frequently piles. This disease if not attended to in time, may terminate in suppuration and abscess, and form fistulous opening by rectum or bladder, or through the peritoneum and thus destroy the life of the patient; or it may remain in the chronic form, which is the most stubborn, obstinate, and most distressful of complaints in the whole category of diseases to treat.

*PROSTATORRHŒA.

Associated with spermatorrhœa we not unfrequently find an excitation of the prostatic and

Cowper's glands, and possibly of the vesiculæ seminales. These glandular structures furnish an increased secretion, having a mucoid appearance, and
slightly resembling seminal fluid, which is passed
with the urine, on going to stool, on lifting or
straining, and in some cases, when profuse, there is
an almost constant oozing. The patient's mind
having been excited by what he has been told by
designing persons, calling themselves physicians, or
by the private circulars he has received from the
same source, he is constantly troubled by it, so
much so that he is not unfrequently on the verge of
insanity.

Not only do we find this discharge in those who
truly have spermatorrhœa, but quite as frequently
when that disease does not exist, the prostatorrhœa
being the only trouble.

The sufferer has, however, been told that he is
suffering from the former affection, and religiously
believes it, the influence on the mind being such as
to frequently impair the general health. It is useless sometimes in these cases to attempt to persuade
them of the mistake in the nature of the disease, so
firmly is it fastened upon their minds; and when
we arrest the discharge we oftentimes get credit for
curing a case of spermatorrhœa.

VARICOCELE.

This disease is frequently met with. It generally
arrives soon after puberty, but occasionally it occurs

later. It consists in a dilated and tortuous state of the veins of the spermatic chord. The disease as a rule is confined to the left side, from the fact that the left spermatic vein is unprovided with a valve, whereas one exists distinctly on the right side.

The causes of this affection are venereal excesses, masturbation, and its effect—constant relaxtion of the scrotum, riding on horseback, pressure on the spermatic vessels from distension of the iliac portion of the colon, tumors in the groin or pelvis, and the wearing of ill-constructed trusses.

It is usually slow in its progress, and at first gives rise to but little disturbance, except a feeling of weight and dragging in the groin. As the veins enlarge, however, the patient suffers aching and dragging pains in the parts, much increased by being upon the feet, by walking, or riding. In some rare cases it causes venereal excitement, but in the majority it lessens it, and often times proves a cause of impotence.

When the disease is fully developed, the veins are convoluted, knotty, elongated, harder in some places than in others, and irregularly dilated. Their walls are very thick, dense, and rigid at some points, and very brittle and attenuated at others.

The tumor resulting from these enlarged and dilated veins is of an elongated, conical shape, irregular and compressible, feeling very much like a bundle of cords, or a cluster of earth-worms.

HYDROCELE.

This is a collection of fluid within the *tunica va-ginalis,* a serous membrane, lining the cavity of the scrotum, having a visceral layer investing the testes, and a reflected layer lining the scrotum. The more common causes of this complaint are such as cause irritation and subsequent enfeeblement of the serous membranes. The fluid which forms the hydrocele is usually transparent and of an amber, pale yellow, and resembles the serum of the blood, but it sometimes becomes quite thick and contains considerable flocculent material, or may even be puru-lent.

The swelling commences in the lower portion of the scrotum, and as the fluid increases gradually extends up to the abdominal ring, pressure does not produce pain, except it is brought to bear upon the testicle, and then there is pain with a sense of faint-ness. The tumor is pyriform in shape, and gives the sensation of a bladder filled with water, with sometimes distinct, sometimes obscure fluctuation.

INCONTINENCE OF URINE.

This trouble, the power of not being able to hold the urine, may occur at any period of life. It may be excited by a great variety of circumstances, among the most prominent of which are masturba-tion, ill-health, external injuries, paralysis, morbid sensibility of the bladder and urethra, stricture, &c. It often begins very early in life in both sexes, and occasionally continues long after the age of puberty, greatly to the annoyance, both physical and mental, of the poor sufferer. The discharge, which may take place several times during the night, is most common toward morning, and is sometimes effected under the influence of the will or of a dream, but, in general, it is strictly involuntary. The discharge may be copious and abundant in a full emission, or may dribble away in drops. The latter is the more common result from stricture and from morbid sensibility of the neck of the bladder induced by masturbation.

In young children it is often produced by ill-health, arising from improper feeding and want of good air and exercise, followed by disorder of the digestive organs; by malarious diseases; by worms in the alimentary canal; by the inordinate use of saccharine drinks; and by the irritating properties or the excessive quantity of the urine.

INFLAMMATION OF THE KIDNEYS.

Inflammation of the kidney may be acute or chronic, the latter being by far the more frequent of the two.

The most common exciting causes are external injury, the presence of renal calculi, irritating diuretics, stricture of the urethra, enlargement of the prostate gland, and chronic disease of the bladder. In some cases it is provoked by the gouty or rheumatic diathesis. The inflammation may be limited to the proper renal tissue, or it may at the same time involve the pelvis of the kidney, thus constituting what is termed *pyelitis.* The most prominent symptoms of *acute nephritis* are sharp, spasmodic, or dull, heavy, deep-seated, aching pains in the loins, increased by pressure and motion, and extending along the spermatic cord, up the back, down the thigh, and into the pelvis; retraction of the testicles; scanty, high-colored urine, which, when tested, is found to contain albumen usually in considerable, and frequently in great abundance; irritability of the bladder, with a frequent desire to micturate; pyrexia, great thirst, restlessness, nausea, vomiting, and, in most cases, constipation of the bowels. The skin becomes dry. Co-incident with this febrile movement there is œdema. It is generally first observed on the face, particularly below the eyes, but it is speedily observed in the lower extremities, and sometimes occurs first in the latter situation. This dropsy sometimes takes place into the peritoneal and pleural cavity and oftentimes occurs to such an extent as to occasion great suffering from dyspnœa, and endanger life. If the urine be examined with the microscope, blood, pus, and renal casts may generally be detected. If permitted to progress, the disease either passes into suppuration, or it assumes the chronic form.

CHRONIC INFLAMMATION OF THE KIDNEYS.

Chronic *nephritis* is generally dependent upon organic disease of the urethra, bladder, or prostate gland, attended with permanent obstructions to the free evacuation of the urine. In consequence of the obstacle thus occasioned, the ureters are habitually distended with urine, and are eventually transformed into subsidiary reservoirs, in which the fluid accumulates in such a manner as to produce serious pressure upon the renal tissues, and ultimately their partial, if not complete, destruction.

The suffering in chronic nephritis is usually much milder than in the acute form. The pain is less severe, and seldom extends to any distance among the neighboring structures ; there is no retraction of the testicles ; the bladder is irritable and impatient of its contents; as a rule there is general dropsy and albumenuria. Frequently the quantity of albumen is large, but this by no means holds true in all cases ; the quantity of albumen is sometimes quite small, and sometimes it does not exist. As a rule, general dropsy is marked in the cases in which the albumen in the urine is very abundant, and, per contra, general dropsy is slight or wanting in the cases in which the urine contains but little albumen or none whatever. The general health, perhaps long impaired, gradually declines, the patient losing flesh, sleep, appetite, and strength. By and by hectic fever sets in, attended with frequent fits of headache, drowsiness, and vomiting, and life is finally worn out by sheer exhaustion. Sometimes death is caused by suppression of urine, preceded and accompanied by coma and convulsions ; at other times, by the sudden supervention of acute nephritis, an event generally announced by rigors, violent fever, and delirium, with great increase of the local distress.

DIABETES INSIPIDUS.

This is an excessive discharge of almost colorless urine, of light weight, containing neither sugar nor albumen. This excessive urination is probably the result of dilatation of the capillary vessels of the kidneys; this having its origin in some remote agency which disturbs the ganglio-nervous influence which controls the circulation.

The causes of the disease are various, and somewhat obscure. Blows on the head, intemperance, cerebral disease, and exposure to cold or drinking cold fluids while heated, are among the supposed causes.

The duration of the complaint varies from a few weeks to many years—or a lifetime. Often beginning suddenly, the amount of water passed may reach ten or twenty quarts *per diem.* Thirst is intense, and withholding liquids does not arrest the excessive discharge. The skin becomes dry and harsh. Debility and emaciation attend, if the attack is prolonged.

DIABETES MELLITUS.

This is excessive urination, with the presence of sugar in the urine. The diuresis is generally a notable feature of the affection, but the presence of grape sugar or glucose in the urine, however, is the distinctive feature of this affection. Sugar in the urine like albumenuria, occurs not unfrequently as a symptom in various pathological connections. The sugar, under these circumstances, is usually not abundant, and the urine contains it for a brief period only. As the distinctive feature of an individual affection, the sugar which the urine contains is in greater or less abundance, and it continues persistingly in the urine. Even when the affection exists the saccharine urine is, in fact, merely a symptom. It does not constitute the affection. It is incidental to, or an effect of, the real disease. The sugar exists in the urine because it pre-exists in the blood. Existing everywhere in the vascular system, it is excreted by the kidneys. But, with our present knowledge, the true seat and nature of the disease are not clearly established. The exciting causes appear to be, exposure to cold and wet, drinking cold water largely when heated, excessive use of saccharine food, intemperance, violent emotion, febrile diseases, and organic affections and injuries of the brain and spinal cord. The disease begins insidiously, with malaise and slight loss of flesh; urination becomes excessive, with corresponding thirst, and very often excessive appetite; emaciation sets in and is progressive; the skin becomes harsh and dry; the tongue is glazed and furrowed, and the mouth clammy; the sexual and mental powers fail by degress. Lastly, hectic fever, œdema of the limbs, diarrhœa, and often all the symptoms of pulmonary consumption terminate the case.

LITHIASIS.

Lithiasis or gravel consists in the formatian of calculous deposits in the kidneys or bladder. These concretions are generally formed within the renal cavities. Calculi of small size may pass from the kidneys to the bladder, giving rise to little or no inconvenience, and having reached the bladder, they are either discharged with the urine, or remaining in the bladder, they increase in size and require for their removal surgical interference. Calculi occasion more or less pain in their passage from the renal cavity, through the ureter, to the bladder in proportion to their size, and the roughness of their surfaces. The pain begins as the calculus enters the duct and ends when it reaches the bladder. These paroxysms of pain are usually developed suddenly, though there is generally more or less sense of uneasiness, due to irritation caused by the presence of the calculi in the pelvis of the kidney. In the male the pain is generally felt in the testicle which is drawn upward by the contraction of the cremaster muscle. It is sometimes so excessive as to force the patient to groan and cry aloud, There is frequent or constant desire to micturate, with the passing of only a few drops at a time. Not unfrequently the urine is bloody. With these local symptoms are associated those denoting more or less constitutional disturbance ; thirst, nausea, and vomiting, coldness of the surface with sweating, and feebleness of the circulation. The countenance is pallid and expressive of anguish. The bowels are usually constipated. Suddenly the pain ceases and the paroxysm ends. The calculus has reached the bladder. An abundant discharge of urine takes place, which may contain the calculi, and more or less purulent or muco-purulent matter.

Not unfrequently concretions varying in size from that of a pin's head to a small pea, pass without giving rise to sufficient pain to constitute a paroxysm.

The composition of the concretions varies in different cases.

The most frequent form of gravel is that in which the concretions consist of uric acid. The discharges being usually of a red color, this variety is sometimes distinguished as red gravel. The concretions may consist of the earthy salts, the ammonio-phosphate of magnesia, phosphate of lime, and the carbonate of lime. The color of these is usually either grayish or white. In another variety the concretions consist of the oxalate of lime. These are of a yellow, brownish or dark color.

INDEX.